Cancer Doesn't Have to Hurt

A Bill of Rights for People with Cancer Pain

- You have the right to have pain relieved by health professionals, family, friends and others around you.

- Your comfort is an important part of health. Pain relief should be treated as a priority.

- You have the right to have pain controlled, no matter what its cause or how severe it may be.

- You have the right to be treated with respect at all times.

- Appropriate use of pain medications is not drug abuse. It is legal and important to your treatment.

- You have the right to have pain caused by procedures and treatments prevented or at least minimized.

- You have a responsibility to help manage your pain.

(From the Iowa Cancer Pain Relief Initiative and the Wisconsin Cancer Pain Initiative. Used with permission.)

Dedication

This book is dedicated to those who suffer from unrelieved cancer pain in the hope that we can make a difference in the quality of your lives, and especially to the memory of Lloyd A. Haylock, Jr., Cynthia Shanahan Anderson, and Marjorie R. Perry.

Cancer Doesn't Have to Hurt

How to Conquer the Pain Caused by Cancer and Cancer Treatment

Pamela J. Haylock, R.N., M.A., E.T.
&
Carol P. Curtiss, R.N., M.S.N., O.C.N.

Hunter House
PUBLISHERS

Library of Congress Cataloging-in-Publication Data
Haylock, Pamela J.
Cancer doesn't have to hurt : how to conquer the pain caused by cancer and cancer treatment / Pamela J. Haylock and Carol P. Curtiss.
p. cm.
Includes bibliographical references and index.
ISBN 0-89793-214-5 (cloth). — ISBN 0-89793-213-7 (pbk.)
1. Cancer pain.   I. Curtiss, Carol P. II. Title.
RC262. H395 1996
616.99'4—dc20   96-18194
CIP

Ordering
Hunter House books are available at bulk discounts for textbook/course adoptions; to qualifying community, healthcare, and government organizations; and for special promotions and fundraising. For details please contact:

Special Sales Department
Hunter House Inc., PO Box 2914, Alameda CA 94501-0914
Tel. (510) 865-5282 Fax (510) 865-4295
e-mail: marketing@hunterhouse.com

Individuals can order our books from most bookstores or by calling toll-free:
1-800-266-5592

Cover Design: MIG/Design Works   Book Design: *Qalagraphia*
Project Editor: Lisa E. Lee   Copy Editor: Mali Apple
Book Production: Paul J. Frindt, Kiran S. Rana, Wendy Low
Editorial Assistance: Kim A. Wallace, Jane E. Moore, Dana Weissman
Proofreader: Lee Rappold   Indexer: Janis Paris
Marketing: Corrine M. Sahli   Promotion: Enver M. Casimir
Customer support: Christina Arciniega, Edgar M. Estavilla, Jr.
Order fulfillment: A & A Quality Shipping Services
Publisher: Kiran S. Rana

Typeset in Aldine 401 BT with titles in Egyptian by Hunter House Inc.
Printed and bound by Publishers Press, Salt Lake City, UT
Manufactured in the United States of America
9 8 7 6 5 4 3 2 1   First edition

Contents

Foreword

by Susan Leigh, R.N., B.S.N., past president, National Coalition for Cancer Survivorship

Pain, unhappily, is an intimate acquaintance of cancer survivors.
Moreover, the diagnosis of cancer often carries the expectation of pain,
bodily distress, and physical suffering such that pain and the fear
of pain often become tangled elements of the burden borne
by the survivor.

— *Fitzhugh Mullan*

Almost everyone who is diagnosed with cancer will suffer from some sort of pain, and this is certainly not limited to those who are dying. As a survivor of three different cancer experiences, I remember the pain from surgical incisions, needle sticks, flexible scopes, biopsies, bone marrow aspirations, radiation burns, severe constipation, persistent vomiting, shingles, bladder irritation, spasms, and infections—and these were only the physical pains. Those of us who have experienced disease or treatment-related pain know that the discomfort, no matter how severe, affects not only our bodies but our minds, our souls, our relationships, our work, our play, and our dreams of the future. Combine physical pain with the emotional pains of fear, vulnerability, and sadness; the social pains of family disruptions, relationship problems, and work and financial concerns; and the spiritual or existential pain of a loss of hope, a threatened lifespan, or a questioning of one's religious beliefs, and the suffering is magnified.

Some pain is temporary, like a needle stick, and we bite the bullet and get through it. Other pain lingers for weeks or months and can drain us of physical, mental, and emotional energy. To alleviate bodily pain, doctors have routinely prescribed medication; nurses have often decided how well the medicine is working; and both doctor and nurse, and sometimes family members, have occasionally judged how much pain we should tolerate. Also, many of us still believe that pain is part of the package, something to be expected and tolerated, while the fear of addiction has mistakenly led to years of uncontrolled suffering. The energy used to fight the pain takes away from that which is needed to heal our bodies and nourish our relationships. While the passive, stoic, and uncomplaining person was in the past described as a "good patient," we can all surely be thankful that society's ideas about bearing pain are changing.

As we become more informed medical consumers, we accept greater responsibility for decisions surrounding our health care. It has become more acceptable to request, and sometimes demand, adequate pain control, and thus we become our own advocates. Yet as cancer survivor and advocate Ellen Hermanson wrote, "you can't expect tired, frightened, and sick patients to do all the work in achieving control over their pain." In order to fight pain with everything at our disposal—medications, complementary therapies, information, communication—we need a good relationship with our health care team and the self-confidence to make our needs known.

This book reminds me of a comprehensive yet easy-to-read *Whole Earth Catalog* for pain management. The authors first recognize pain as a major health problem and then help us to understand this symptom in relation to cancer. They emphasize our right to pain control, offer us practical tools to identify and describe our experience, and help take the mystery out of managing our distress by exploring both mainstream medicine and complementary therapies.

While valuable resources are listed, an important message

within these pages reminds us to recognize how different we all are as individuals. We will all react to pain in very different ways. Just as our cancers are different, so too are our physical and emotional health, circumstances, cultures, and the meanings we give to pain. To use the resources available to us and to make pain manageable, we must learn to find the right words and to adequately describe our suffering.

When we do begin to put pain into language, it begins to tell a story, and that story often diminishes or erases pain. So the effort to find a language for pain is both important and healing.

— *M. Lerner*

By teaching us the language of pain, the authors help us to rewrite our scripts and to design our destinies. May this book help all your stories have happier endings.

References

Hermanson, E. 1994. In Pursuit of Pain Relief: A Survivor's Story. *The NCCS Networker* 8(4), 3.

Lerner, M. 1994. *Choices in Healing: Integrating the Best of Conventional and Complementary Approaches to Cancer.* Cambridge, Mass.: The MIT Press, 472.

Mullan, F., M.D. Statement on behalf of the National Coalition for Cancer Survivorship on the occasion of the release of the *Clinical Practice Guideline on the Management of Cancer Pain,* March 2, 1994.

A Message from the Authors

We have both been nurses for over twenty-five years. Most of that time, we have specialized in caring for people and families facing cancer. We have seen great progress in how cancer is managed. In spite of that progress, people with cancer still suffer with pain. We know that *cancer doesn't have to hurt*—that most of the pain of cancer and cancer treatment is unnecessary. Doctors, nurses, and even the person with pain can be blamed for this needless suffering. These same people can make pain go away. Since all doctors, nurses, and pharmacists may not be skilled in cancer pain control, the person with cancer—and his or her family—have to demand that pain be controlled. Health care professionals are slowly but surely learning how to do this. The United States government has issued formal advice for treating cancer pain. Special classes help nurses, pharmacists, and doctors learn to manage cancer pain better.

We want this book to give people facing cancer the facts in words that are easy to understand. Scientific studies reveal that people who have trouble describing pain and those whose knowledge about pain is minimal are the people who have the most pain. We know that knowledge is power, and we want people facing cancer to have the power to get pain under control. This is our purpose for and hope in writing this book.

In the book, we often refer to "the patient" even though we realize that some people with cancer or cancer survivors dislike this term—preferring instead to be designated as "survivor." In written materials, the Oncology Nursing Press often replaces the word "patient" with "the person with cancer." We elect to refer to the "person with cancer" and "cancer survivor" simply as "patient" and hope readers will accept this use as an attempt at clarity.

The absence of pain helps people live better, and there are now signs that the absence of pain also helps people live longer. There are treatments and methods that can relieve most pain caused by cancer. Almost everyone can find ways to ease cancer-related pain. This book will help you find comfort for yourself or someone you care for.

Acknowledgements

The authors gratefully acknowledge the support, encouragement, and assistance provided by Carol Blecher, R.N., C.C.N.S., A.O.C.N., M.S.; Barbara Britt, R.N., M.S.N.; Betty Ferrell, Ph.D., R.N., F.A.A.N.; Margaret Gosselin, Ed.D.; Susan Leigh, R.N., B.S.N.; Anne Sasaki, M.S.W.; and Don D. Wilson, M.D. We are particularly indebted to the many people with cancer and their families who have taught us so much.

We appreciate our publisher, Hunter House, and especially thank Mali Apple, our copy editor, for helping us put our words down in ways that the reader can easily use; Lisa Lee, project manager and editor, for her enthusiasm for the idea of "Cancer Doesn't Have to Hurt"; Jenny Moore, editorial coordinator, for helping us collaborate with each other and Hunter House despite distance; and Kiran Rana, publisher, for giving us this opportunity to reach more people than we ever could in our usual day-to-day lives.

With thanks and love to Don, Jack, Jennifer, and Paul.

Introduction

Key Points

- Cancer doesn't have to hurt.

- Everyone has a right to demand good control of pain.

- The barriers to good control of cancer pain can be conquered by knowledge.

Over half of all people diagnosed with cancer are treated successfully. Many who cannot be cured can live with their cancers under control for quite a while—some for many years. It doesn't matter if the aim of treatment is cure, control or comfort: all people with cancer should expect to enjoy whatever time they have no matter how long or short. For many, effective pain control is key.

Pain is a thief. Pain robs the person in pain of the chance to enjoy being alive—the chance to go on a picnic, go to a family dinner, or take a pleasant walk. Pain robs a child of good times with a parent or grandparent. Pain makes it hard to get dressed in the morning and to do other things we all take for granted. Fixing meals, eating, or even talking can be a challenge for someone in pain. Severe pain makes it hard to sleep and impossible to work. Pain can cause a person to make big changes in his or her day-to-day life. Pain causes some people to withdraw from friends and relatives. In fact, most people say they don't really fear death from cancer: what they really fear is the pain they believe goes hand in hand with cancer.

For many people with cancer, "pain relief takes a lot of energy. Pain relief can take a long time to get it right,...but time, for many of us, is a problem." So says Ellen Hermanson, a seven-year breast cancer survivor. Ms. Hermanson goes on to say she learned that pain control is a balancing act and that the balance can change almost daily.

People with cancer have a right to comfort. This right is expressed in the "Bill of Rights for People with Cancer Pain" which begins below. Professional organizations like the Oncology Nursing Society, the American Cancer Society, the American Pain Society, and the American Society of Clinical Oncologists agree. The American court system recognizes this right too. In 1990, a North Carolina court awarded $15 million to the family of a man with cancer who died in pain in a nursing home where he was not given pain control medicines. The responsibility to provide good pain control is clear. Doctors, nurses, pharmacists, and people with cancer pain are partners in controlling cancer pain.

People with cancer do not have to be in severe pain. People with cancer pain have the right to have pain treated aggressively. Relieving cancer pain is the responsibility of every person caring for people with cancer. Professional organizations like the Oncology Nursing Society, state cancer pain initiatives, and the American Society of Clinical Oncology concur: health care providers have an ethical duty to try everything possible to relieve cancer pain. Unrelieved pain increases suffering and the burden of having cancer. Failing to treat cancer pain is not acceptable medical or nursing practice. But still, many people remain in pain needlessly.

A Bill of Rights for People with Cancer Pain

- You have the right to have pain relieved by health professionals, family, friends and others around you.

- Your comfort is an important part of health. Pain relief should be treated as a priority.

- You have the right to have pain controlled, no matter what its cause or how severe it may be.

- You have the right to be treated with respect at all times.

- Appropriate use of pain medications is not drug abuse. It is legal and important to your treatment.

- You have the right to have pain caused by procedures and treatments prevented or at least minimized.

- You have a responsibility to help manage your pain.

(From the Iowa Cancer Pain Relief Initiative and the Wisconsin Cancer Pain Initiative. Used with permission.)

If we know how to treat cancer pain, why do so many suffer? Pain control has not improved much in spite of better education; knowing what to do does not always mean doing it right. C. Stratton Hill, M.D., in a December 20, 1995, editorial in the *Journal of the American Medical Association,* writes, "Significant change regarding pain control may depend on empowering patients to demand adequate pain treatment." One goal of this book is to help readers know what to expect and what to ask for. Demand adequate pain control. Do not be satisfied with less. Life is too important to suffer needlessly.

Attitudes & Knowledge

Our attitudes toward pain and our knowledge of how to control pain have a great effect on our efforts to control pain. This is true for doctors, nurses, pharmacists, and social workers as well as for people with cancer and their family members or friends.

Attitudes

An attitude is a frame of mind based on a set of beliefs. What we accept as true about pain and cancer pain comes from what we have felt or seen in our lives. If you see that most people with cancer have pain, then you will come to believe that pain is an unavoidable effect of cancer. If this is your belief, you will be less likely to think that pain control is possible and, therefore, less likely to ask for better pain relief. The belief that pain always follows cancer is a block to good pain control.

Faulty ideas about the medicines used to control pain also affect the ability of caregivers to help a person in pain. A fear of addiction keeps many people from using medicines like codeine or morphine. Some people believe that these medicines will lose their ability to control pain if they are used "too much," so they save the medicines for later when the pain gets "really bad." Such myths get in the way of good pain relief. Chapter 8 explains the truth about addiction and tolerance and their relation to pain-relieving medicines.

Knowledge

Many doctors, nurses, pharmacists, and other health care professionals have new skills that allow good treatment of cancer pain. But for others, outdated ideas and beliefs get in the way. Some doctors and nurses have very little schooling in managing cancer pain. They may be unaware of new information and standards that guide cancer pain control. Even some who are aware of new information do not change their practices when it comes to cancer pain relief.

For people with cancer pain, some of the basic keys to controlling that pain may seem strange at first. For example, most of us will take pain medicine when we have pain. But taking pain medicine on a schedule, even when we don't have pain, is a new idea—but it is vital to good pain control. Long-held beliefs often get in the way of good pain relief.

Asking questions of the doctor or nurse is not easy for many people. Many people think the doctor or nurse will know about the pain without being told. The doctor or nurse might assume that you will let them know if you are having pain. When neither the health care professional nor the person with pain brings up the subject of pain, it may never be properly treated.

Cost

Pain can be costly. Pain causes many people to miss work, and that costs money. Missing work causes some people to lose insurance coverage or, worse still, their jobs. Most of us will go to great lengths to be free of pain. This might mean spending money—in some cases, lots of money. The cost of pain-relieving drugs taken by mouth, by far the most common and effective treatment, often runs close to $100 each month. Other methods cost more. Pain-control costs may be more than one can pay. Depending on whether a person has insurance and on the type of insurance coverage she or he has, payment for pain medications may or may not be covered. In fact, many insurance policies, including Medicare, don't cover the cost of prescription medicines except those used during a hospital stay or doctor's office visit.

Pain is big business. In some respects this is good, as more focus is put on pain control. More people involved in pain control means more information about, more progress in, and more access to pain control. Good cancer care and good pain control can be found in cities, towns, and even rural communities.

A drawback of the "business of pain" is that new procedures and products can be extremely costly. For example, some companies design machines used to give pain control medicines. Costs for the machine, the nurse, pharmacist, or doctor who monitors or assists with its use, and the supplies needed to run it can range from $2,000 to $5,000 each month. Some of these "high tech" methods are covered by some insurance policies. Unfortunately, new devices and techniques sometimes become almost routine before they are proven to be better than older, easier, and less costly methods of pain control.

Laws and Regulations

Some lawmakers believe that legally prescribed medicines too often make their way to other people. This "diversion" for illegal use of prescribed medicines is, according to these lawmakers, a big part of America's drug problem. Pain experts disagree. Instead, they believe that laws and regulations that protect against diversion limit access to these medicines for people who truly need them.

Most laws and regulations that cover the major painkilling medicines are enacted by the states and vary from state to state. State laws govern how many pills a doctor can write for with each prescription and how many prescriptions for analgesic opioids a physician can write each month. Regulations restrict some doctors from prescribing these medicines at all. State regulations guide how some of these medicines are to be stored in local pharmacies, and whether a local pharmacy even can sell them.

This book will discuss these and many other issues affecting cancer pain and its treatment—and will help people with cancer and their family and friends to take control of cancer pain.

Cancer and Pain

Key Points

- Good cancer care involves taking care of pain.

- The best treatment for pain is treatment that takes into account the cause of pain.

- Pain can be directly caused by cancer in many ways.

- Pain can be caused by cancer treatment.

- Pain can be caused by the side effects of cancer treatment.

- Regardless of the cause of pain, pain can be relieved.

The International Association for the Study of Pain defines pain as "an unpleasant sensory and emotional experience associated with actual or potential tissue damage or described in terms of such damage."

The pain that people with cancer have can be caused by one or many problems. Pain can occur when a tumor presses on nerves or organs. The "poking and prodding" that happens when cancer is being diagnosed can be uncomfortable and sometimes painful. Cancer treatment—surgery, the actual treatment, and side effects of treatment—can be painful. Pain can be a symptom of infections that occur as a result of the cancer or cancer treatment. Finally, the cancer process can cause other problems that produce pain.

Cancer pain experts divide pain into two major types, defined by the cause of the pain and how the sensation of pain reaches the brain. *Nociceptive* pain is caused by tissue damage. *Neuropathic* pain occurs when nerves themselves are affected or damaged. Nociceptive and neuropathic pain affect people in different ways and is managed in different ways.

Nociceptive pain is often easy to describe and to locate. Most people describe it using words like "sharp," "ache," "throbbing," or "pressure." It is common for people with neuropathic pain to use words like "shooting," "sharp," "burning," "tight," "constricting," "numbness," "fullness," or "heaviness" to describe their pain. Sometimes, people with neuropathic pain have areas of extreme tenderness at specific parts of their bodies.

Cancer-Related Problems That Cause Pain

Nociceptive pain occurs when cancer spreads to bone, muscle, organs, and joints. The cancer can spread just by growing larger in its original or "primary" area. Or, cancer cells can break away from the primary tumor and enter the bloodstream or lymph system and reach other areas of the body in what is called *metastatic* spread. Pain is often a symptom of blockage of an organ or body system, such as a blocked colon (large intestine), small bowel (small intestines), or other parts of the digestive system like the bile ducts, liver, or gall bladder. Pain might also hint at an obstruction in the windpipe (trachea) or bronchi, the major passage from the windpipe to the lungs. When blood vessels or lymph vessels are blocked by a tumor, pain occurs as a result of the swelling (edema).

Bone pain

The most common cause of pain in people with cancer is metastatic bone disease, caused when cancer spreads to bone. Usually, long bones, like the bones in the upper arm and upper leg, and major bones, like those in the pelvis, hips, and spine (vertebrae), are the targets of metastatic disease. Even so, sometimes a tumor spreads to the ribs, shoulder, scapula (shoulder blade), clavicle (collar bone), sternum (breastbone), and the skull.

The cancer cells in these sites cause the body to start a process—a reaction to the invasion by the cancer cells—that leads to the feeling of pain. Pain may be felt at the actual place where a tumor has spread to the bone. The pain may also be "referred" to a distant body area, meaning that it may be felt in a part of the body that seems far away from the spot where the cancer cells are. For example, people whose cancer has spread to the hip might experience knee pain. Those with cancer spreading to the lower spine might have pain that seems to shoot down the back of one or both legs. Referred pain is the result of the natural pathway of the body's nerves. In fact, people can feel pain in several places at once.

Nerve Pain

Neuropathic pain occurs when nerves are damaged. It can be the result of a tumor pressing on or invading a nerve, a group of nerves, or the spinal cord. In *plexopathy*, pain is produced when a tumor puts pressure on a bundle of nerves called the *plexus*. The most common of these involve nerves around the neck, the arm, and the lower back. Pain coming from the plexus in the neck area (*cervical plexus*) is often described as an ache that spreads or radiates into the neck and the lower back of the skull. Pain coming from another plexus in the neck area (*brachial plexus*) is most often found in people with breast cancer, lung cancer, and lymphoma, a cancer involving the lymph cells. It can also be caused by a metastatic tumor. Most people with tumors involving the brachial plexus experience this type of pain. Depending on how the plexus is involved in the cancer, this type of pain can start in the shoulder and feel like a shooting pain or an electrical shock in the thumb and index finger. Or, the pain can start in the shoulder and radiate down the elbow, arm, and middle forearm, into the ring and little fingers.

Pain Caused by Pressure from Tumors

Pressure on the spinal cord from a primary or metastatic tumor can cause both pain and increasing degrees of numbness and paralysis. This is called *spinal cord compression* and is treated as an emergency. Pain, even slight pain, may be the first sign of this problem. Generally, the pain will slowly increase over a period of weeks until signs of paralysis appear. Other signs of spinal cord compression include changes in bowel or bladder function (constipation, loss of control of bowels and urine). Spinal cord compression is most common in people with cancers of the breast, prostate, or lung. Multiple myeloma (a cancer of the plasma cells), renal cell (kidney) cancer, and melanoma (a form of skin cancer) are often linked to spinal cord compression. Pain is located along the backbone. If nerves are involved, the pain may be described as "sharp" and "shooting."

For most people, spinal cord compression is diagnosed with a simple x-ray of the spine. When pain is assessed and treatment started early, permanent disability can be prevented.

Cord compression is treated with steroids (to decrease swelling around the spinal cord), radiation therapy, and, less often, surgery. Pain control is needed regardless of the form of treatment, but the requirements for pain medicine will decrease if the treatment is successful.

Pain Related to Treatment of Cancer

Whenever possible, the best treatment for pain directly caused by a tumor includes cancer treatment. Surgery can be an option to relieve pressure in cases where a tumor can be reduced in size or removed. Radiation and chemotherapy are also used to reduce the size of a tumor and relieve obstruction. Pain control will be an important part of cancer treatment until pain is gone. If treating the cancer is not an option, pain-relieving medicines will play a major role in providing comfort.

Many of the cancer treatment methods used today can cause pain. Side effects or long-term effects of treatment can result in various kinds of pain as well.

Surgery

The cancer treatment most likely to cause pain is surgery. The pain from an operation usually goes away as the incision heals, but this is not always the case. Sometimes the internal scars left by surgery can interfere with the function of nerves, resulting in pain. A rare pain problem called *reflex sympathetic dystrophy* occurs in some people who have had surgery for lung cancer. Blood vessels that supply blood to nerves are affected, causing coldness of the affected arm, hand, leg, or foot; whiteness or "blanching" when the area is pressed; and severe pain when the skin is barely touched. In serious cases the affected limb does not function at all. Table 1 lists some types of surgery with related signs and symptoms of pain.

The pain problems that occur after surgery are of two types. First, there is the pain that comes from the incision and the surgery itself. This "acute" pain is fairly simple to manage, and most people know that this pain won't last. The acute pain that comes from surgery is managed with strong opioids—the same medicines used to manage chronic pain and cancer pain. Less severe acute pain can be controlled with medicines like acetaminophen (e.g. Tylenol), ibuprofen (e.g. Advil) and weaker opioids like codeine. *Patient-controlled analgesia (PCA)*, a system that allows the patient to control his or her own medicine for pain, is very useful for people recovering from surgery. In fact, PCA was first used for surgical patients before its value in treating cancer pain was known. (For more about PCA, see Chapter 4.)

Pain from long-term effects of surgery is not as easy to manage. The success of pain control in this case depends on knowing whether the pain is from nerve damage or from other body changes caused by the surgery. Table 1 (page 14) lists common cancer operations and related long-term (chronic) pain problems.

Chemotherapy

Many people are not bothered by the needles used to give chemotherapy, while others cannot tolerate the pain of several "sticks" when the IV is started. For people who will get several cycles of chemotherapy, perhaps over several months' time, some doctors and nurses recommend having a *vascular access device* inserted. These devices vary in shape, size, and function. Some are special tubes, or catheters, that are inserted through the skin and tunneled just under the skin to reach a major blood vessel. Another vascular access device,

Table 1: Pain After Cancer Operations

Surgery	Signs and Symptoms
Radical neck dissection (for cancers of the head and neck)	Tight, burning sensation in the neck Numbness or prickly sensations in the neck
Mastectomy (for breast cancer)	Tight, constricting, burning pain in the back of the arm, the armpit, and over the chest; pain is worse when the arm is moved Swelling of the arm (lymphedema) that happens even after lumpectomy when lymph nodes in the armpit are damaged
Thoracotomy (for lung cancer)	Ache along the scar Loss of feeling around the scar Extreme tenderness at certain points along the scar Reflex sympathetic dystrophy may develop
Nephrectomy (removal of a kidney)	Numbness, fullness, or heaviness in the side, front of the abdomen, and groin
Amputation of a leg or arm	Phantom limb pain (often happens when there was pain in the site before the amputation) Stump pain can occur over the scar several months to years after surgery Burning sensation that is made worse by movement

(Adapted from Agency for Health Care Policy and Research. Clinical practice guideline no. 9. *Management of Cancer Pain*. Rockville, Md.: U.S. Department of Health and Human Services, March 1994.)

called a port, is a very small container attached to a long catheter (see Figure 1). The port is placed under the skin in a minor operation usually done on an outpatient basis. The tube is attached to the port at one end; the other end is threaded through a blood vessel into one of the large veins that enters the heart.

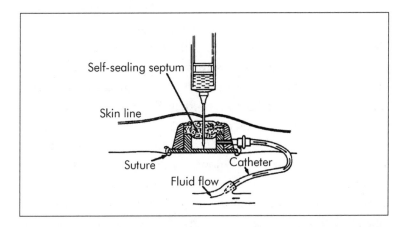

Figure 1: An Implanted Port Access Device. A needle inserted through the skin into the port is attached to a syringe or an IV line. Medicine and fluids can be given through the port. (Reprinted with permission from Winters, V. Implantable vascular access devices. *Oncology Nursing Forum* 11(6):25–30, 1984.)

With the port in place, all that is needed to access a vein to give chemotherapy is a single needle stick that most people find causes only a bit of discomfort. Ports are also used to draw blood for the many blood tests most cancer patients need. Having a port placed is something everyone about to begin chemotherapy should discuss with the doctor or nurse.

The most common side effects of chemotherapy are nausea and vomiting. While some people might not think of this as true pain, nausea and vomiting are surely unpleasant sensory and emotional experiences and, as such, fall into the larger definition of pain. There are now effective ways to decrease or even stop nausea and vomiting. These methods need to be discussed with the doctor and nurse before chemotherapy treatment is started. Medicines like Kytril, Zofran, Compazine, and Reglan are some of the effective antinausea medicines available.

There are other pain syndromes caused by the side effects of chemotherapy. Some chemotherapy drugs, called *vesicants,* are very harmful to tissues. During chemotherapy, some of the drug can leak out of the vein. This is called *extravasation.* The tissue damage from extravasation can be slight, or it can be severe and very painful. In severe cases, wound care is started and plastic surgery might be needed. Extravasation occurs less often when the nurse or doctor giving the chemotherapy has experience and good skills in giving these medicines. The risk of extravasation has gone down with the use of special IV catheters and access devices. The nurse or doctor can also decrease the chance of extravasation, or at least reduce the chance of severe tissue damage, by asking the patient to mention any burning feeling or pain as the chemotherapy is being given. If extravasation is suspected, certain techniques can be started then and there to stop further tissue damage. Ask if the chemotherapy being used is a vesicant; if it is, ask what you can do to reduce the chance of extravasation.

Another common side effect of chemotherapy is the development of sores inside the mouth, the lining of the throat, and the lining of the intestines. The sores in the mouth and throat are called *"stomatitis."* These sores can be painful and make eating and swallowing liquids very difficult. These sores are also sources of danger for people with cancer for two big reasons: First, when pain interferes with eating and drinking, the person may fail to take in enough food and water. Second, the open sores allow germs to enter the body and cause infection.

Stomatitis is treated with medicines that coat and protect the sores. A thick liquid or syrup that contains an anesthetic—

much like what a dentist uses to numb a part of the mouth before working on a tooth—can be used to coat the mouth before meals and make swallowing less painful. These mixtures may also contain antibiotics that help fight germs that cause infection.

Some kinds of chemotherapy cause sores in the lining of the intestines, called mucositis, which are similar to the sores that form inside the mouth. These sores can cause a person to feel bloated and have cramps and diarrhea. Diarrhea may cause the loss of important fluid and nutrients. Cramps, a bloated feeling, and diarrhea contribute to the loss of appetite that is common for people with cancer. If these symptoms develop, it is important for the doctor prescribing chemotherapy and the nurse administering it to be told. (Of course, they should ask, but sometimes they forget.) There are medicines that can relieve cramps, gas, and diarrhea. If symptoms are severe, chemotherapy might be changed (the type changed or dose lowered) so that these side effects do not become major problems.

Some chemotherapy medicines cause *peripheral neuropathy*, in which the nerves that send sensations from the hands, fingers, feet, and toes are damaged. The damage causes tingling, numbness, pain, and sometimes loss of function in hands, fingers, feet, and toes. The drugs most likely to cause this type of damage are Vincristine, Vinblastine, Cisplatin, and Taxol, particularly when used in high doses and over a long period of time. At this time, there is no way to prevent peripheral neuropathy. It is important to inform the doctor or nurse if these symptoms are present so therapy can be adjusted.

Radiation therapy

Other than the discomfort of lying on a hard table, radiation treatments do not cause pain. However, some of the short- and long-term side effects of radiation can be painful.

Radiation works by damaging cancer cells. Even though there is an attempt to protect normal tissue (like skin and the inside of the mouth), radiation damages both normal and cancer cells. Normal cells have the ability to repair themselves; the damage is not permanent. Cancer cells do not have the ability to repair themselves and die as a result of radiation damage. In general, it is the damage to normal cells and tissues that causes the uncomfortable and painful side effects of radiation therapy.

The different kinds of tissues in our bodies vary in the way they respond to radiation. Some tissues—like the mucous membrane that lines the mouth, the lining of the trachea, and the lining of the intestines—are affected easily and quickly. The reaction of these tissues to radiation can range from dryness to open sores. Skin also reacts in varying degrees, from something that looks (and feels) like a sunburn, to skin dryness and peeling that can cause sores to form. These sores are themselves a source of pain and put the person at high risk for infection. A good skin care program can reduce the chance of having these reactions. The radiation therapy nurse or doctor can offer advice for care of the skin. Most skin care plans include using special lotions or creams. In some treatment centers, aloe vera gel is used to protect the skin. If skin problems do occur, the doctor or nurse needs to give directions for care.

Radiation will affect only the parts of the body that fall within the *treatment field*—the parts that are the target of the beam of radiation. Also, not everyone will develop severe side effects: our abilities to endure treatment vary widely. For example, when the chest is treated after surgery for lung cancer, the parts of the body that *might* develop side effects include the skin, the lung tissue that is exposed to the radiation, the trachea and bronchi that are exposed, and for some people, the lower neck area. Many people will also develop a sore throat and have trouble swallowing. People who have radiation treatment after surgery for colon or rectal cancer might develop diarrhea and skin sores as a result of damage to the skin and the remaining bowel or rectum.

A rare pain syndrome associated with radiation and surgery occurs when scarlike or fibrous tissue forms around a bundle of nerves (a *plexus*) interfering with their function. The result is the same as the plexus pain syndromes described earlier that are directly caused by a tumor (see pages 10–12). Experts say that the plexus pain syndromes caused by radiation are less severe than those caused by tumor. A *brachial* plexus is located in each of the two sides of the lower neck and controls sensations to the hand, arm, upper ribcage, and shoulder. When surgery or radiation therapy involves this area, rigid scar tissue can trap and put pressure on this bundle of nerves. This neuropathic type of pain can be quite severe and difficult, but not impossible, to manage. A combined approach offered by several health care providers, involving a combination of medicines, different ways to take the medicines, and various self-care techniques, offers the best chances for success in these complex cases.

Other Causes of Pain

Fatigue

In addition to direct side effects of cancer and its treatment, there are other causes of pain that relate to cancer and cancer treatment. Fatigue is a common side effect of cancer and cancer treatment. Fatigue can limit the person's ability to get around—to walk or even to move.

Pressure sores

Pressure sores, or bed sores, develop when a person stays in one position too long. The top layers of skin are rubbed away, and the blood vessels between the bone and skin surface are closed off, or crimped. When this happens, blood can't get through to supply the skin and tissue with oxygen. The skin and other tissues die. When the skin is damaged, nerves are exposed and pain occurs. Aside from pain, these open sores provide a place for germs to enter the body and cause infection. Preventing pressure sores is of great importance, as they are painful and difficult to heal. Taking care of a pressure sore involves relieving pressure and keeping the wound clean. Pain can be managed through medication and by keeping the sore—and exposed nerve endings—covered with special dressings. A nurse who is expert at taking care of wounds can be a good source of advice and help for people and families dealing with pressure sores.

Immobility and pneumonia

Lack of motion, or immobility, decreases a person's ability to fully expand the lungs when breathing. Fatigue and immobility can hinder a person's ability to cough. And, when lungs don't expand all the way and the ability to cough is decreased, mucous secretions, or *phlegm,* collect in the lungs and allow germs to grow. Pneumonia develops this way. Drinking enough water and other fluids helps to keep the phlegm thin, and coughing can help get rid of phlegm. Coughing and deep-breathing exercises can help to rid the lungs of the phlegm. Other ways to exercise the lungs include blowing up a balloon or use of an *incentive spirometer* on a regular basis (e.g. every hour). The nurse or respiratory therapist can suggest ways to expand the lungs and prevent pneumonia.

Constipation

Constipation is a common cause of pain. It can be caused by several factors including limited fluid intake, certain medicines, changes in diet, inactivity, surgery, and direct pressure on the colon from a tumor. To some people, constipation might seem like a minor, slightly embarrassing problem, but for others, the pain caused by constipation is serious.

The most important cause of constipation is diet. The lack of fluid and fiber in the diet is a frequent problem for people with cancer. Immobility adds to the problems leading to constipation. Constipation is the most common side effect of opiates (like codeine and morphine), the most effective pain-relieving medicines. It is a side effect of other medicines too, such as medicines used to treat depression, high blood pressure, fluid retention, and heart problems.

Signs of constipation include discomfort or pain in the stomach area, a feeling of distention or fullness, nausea, and even diarrhea. A rectal exam by the doctor or nurse might reveal a hard and dry stool. Hemorrhoids (sometimes called piles) can be aggravated when the person strains to have a bowel movement (BM) or pass the stool. In severe cases, constipation can even be dangerous—causing tears in the bowel and rectum.

Experts demand that a constipation-prevention program be part of any pain control program. Common anticonstipation advice includes four main points:

1. Fluid: Drink eight glasses (about 2 quarts) of water each day. Drink a small glass of fluid upon arising in the morning, with each meal, and between meals. *Do not* substitute coffee, tea, carbonated drinks (or soda), or grapefruit juice for water; these fluids may increase the body's output of urine and actually decrease body fluid.

2. Fiber: Eat at least 6 to 10 grams of fiber each day. Two tablespoons of wheat bran supplies nearly 6 grams of fiber. Good sources of fiber include beans, broccoli, raisins, sweet potatoes, and some fruits and berries (see Table 2). Fiber helps the body retain water and results in softer, bulkier stool. Bulky stool helps stimulate bowel movement.

3. Exercise: Try to increase activity, even if it is just a 30-minute walk each day. Regular exercise stimulates the bowel.

4. Regular toilet routine: For many people, the strongest urge to have a bowel movement occurs after breakfast. Going to the toilet, or just sitting on the commode for a while at this time, can be useful in getting into a regular toilet routine.

Table 2: Dietary Fiber Content of Selected Foods

Food	Amount	Fiber (grams)
Flour, whole meal (100%)	1 cup	11.9
Beans, kidney, cooked	1 cup	9.7
Raspberries, red, raw	1 cup	9.2
Beans, brown, cooked	1 cup	8.4
All bran or 100% bran	1 cup	8.4
Squash, winter, cooked	1 cup	7.0
Blackberries	1 cup	6.7
Spinach, cooked	1 cup	6.5

Food	Amount	Fiber (grams)
Shredded wheat	2 biscuits	5.6
Mango	1 medium	5.8
Flour, oat, whole	1 cup	5.0
Corn, sweet, cooked	1 cup	4.7
Potatoes, sweet, baked	1 medium	4.2
Broccoli, cooked	1 cup	3.5
Strawberries, raw	1 cup	3.1
Peanuts, fresh or roasted	1 ounce	2.7
Apricots	3 medium	2.6
Plums	2 medium	2.4
Blueberries	1 cup	1.9
Nectarine	1 medium	1.8
Walnuts	1 ounce	1.5

(Source: Canty, S. L. Constipation as a side effect of opioids. *Oncology Nursing Forum* 21(4):739–743, 1994.)

Laxatives and stool softeners can help reduce constipation problems (see Table 3). Laxatives induce bowel movement in three ways: (1) they cause fluid to be retained in the colon, (2) they decrease absorption of water from the colon, and (3) they increase the movement of the bowel (peristalsis) that pushes stool toward the rectum and out of the body.

Many experts also recommend the use of senna containing laxatives to prevent the constipation that results from taking opioid pain-relieving medicines. One tablet of senna taken twice a day is a good starting dose. The dose can be adjusted up or down until regular and normal bowel movements occur.

Preventing constipation is a simple matter of combining diet, exercise, and a mild laxative in a bowel program. It is recommended that each person confer with the doctor or nurse to determine a useful anticonstipation program.

Table 3:   Comparison of Common Laxatives

Laxative Type Generic Name	Brand Names	Onset of Action	How It Works	Comments
Saline Epsom salt, Milk of Magnesia, magnesium citrate	Fleets, GoLytely	1/2 hour–3 hours	Retains water in the colon and stimulates bowel action	May affect fluid and electrolyte balance and should not be used routinely
Irritant/ Stimulant Cascara, senna, phenolphthalein, bisacodyl or castor oil	Ex-Lax, Senoket, Agoral, Alophen, Dulcolax	6–10 hours	Directly stimulates the lining of the colon	Castor oil might be the choice if total clearing of the bowel is needed
Bulk-producing Methylcellulose, Phylum, Polycarbophil	Metamucil, Fibercon	12–24 hours (can be up to 72 hours)	Holds water in the stool and increases its size	Safest and most natural laxative

Laxative Type Generic Name	Brand Names	Onset of Action	How It Works	Comments
Lubricant Mineral oil		6–8 hours	Slows loss of water from the stool and softens stool	May decrease absorption of some vitamins
Surfactants	Docusate, Colace, Dialose, Senoket-S	24–72 hours	Mixes fat with water to soften stool	Helpful when feces are hard or dry or when passage of a firm stool is painful
Miscellaneous Glycerin suppository Lactulose	Fleet Constulose, Enulose, Lactulose	15–30 minutes 24–48 hours	Irritates the colon and causes bowel action	

(Source: Canty, S. L. Constipation as a side effect of opioids. *Oncology Nursing Forum* 21(4):739–745, 1994.)

Impaction

Severe constipation that results in a blocked (obstructed) colon is called *impaction*. Impaction is often overlooked, especially in older people. In a report in the *New England Journal of Medicine*, nearly half of all elderly people admitted to a hospital ward had an impaction. Impaction can be diagnosed by a simple rectal exam that finds hard, dry stool in the lower bowel. Sometimes the impaction is higher in the bowel, and an X-ray is needed to locate the blockage.

Serious problems are associated with impaction, including diarrhea (as mucus and stool seep around the impaction), skin breakdown from the diarrhea, infections of the urinary tract, total bowel obstruction, and direct passage of bacteria from the intestine to the urinary bladder. Impaction is treated by removing the hard, dry stool. To do this, a nurse (or a caregiver who has learned how) can insert one or two gloved and lubricated fingers into the rectum to break up and remove the impaction. This is followed by an enema or bisacodyl (Dulcolax) suppository to completely empty the bowel. A regular anticonstipation bowel program should be started and continued as long as factors leading to constipation are present.

People and Pain

Pain means different things to different people. People vary in how they think about pain. In turn, what people think about pain can affect how they react to it. How a person reacts to pain is an important part in making a plan to control pain. Let's consider what pain means.

Some people believe pain is God's way of punishing them for past sins or even bad or sinful thoughts. While proving the truth of this belief is impossible, the belief is common and hard to fight. If a person with pain believes the pain is deserved, he or she might not be willing to work out a pain control plan. Nurses and doctors who work with people in pain witness the fact that cancer pain affects good and bad people. Actual or imagined sins seem to have nothing to do with who has pain and who does not. If a person's religious beliefs seem to have something to do with pain, it might be useful to talk with a minister, priest, rabbi, or other religious advisor.

Culture may set a person's attitude toward pain. Some research suggests that people of different cultural groups think about and react to pain in different ways. People in some groups are more vocal about their pain. People in some groups are more likely to demand pain control. And some groups of people are more likely to try to endure pain.

A person's age and sex might affect his or her thoughts about and reactions to pain. Men and boys in some cultures are expected to be brave and to "tough it out" when it comes to pain. Females and older people are more likely to admit to having pain and be willing to describe it. On the other hand, older people are less likely to admit that they have severe pain.

For many people, pain is a sign that the cancer has spread or that the disease is getting worse. Though this is not always true, if a person with cancer believes this to be the case, he or she can become anxious or depressed. Anxiety and depression need to be taken into account when planning for pain control. For many people, treatment of anxiety and depression are helpful in their overall pain-control plan.

How Pain Affects Family and Friends

Family members and friends of people with cancer say that pain is one of the hardest aspects of coping with the cancer of a loved one. It is very hard to accept that someone we care for is in pain. Knowing someone has pain, and feeling helpless to make it better, adds to the stress and worry of having a friend or family member with cancer.

Some family members and friends react with anger. Or a feeling of helplessness may cause them to avoid visits and telephone calls to the person with cancer. The anger or sadness can also lead to emotional problems for caregivers and make them less able to offer help. Well-meaning family members or friends may try to help but actually do not have either the skills or the knowledge to do the right thing.

Family members and friends can have a good deal of influence on how a person expresses and copes with their pain. For example, if family members and friends believe that pain can be relieved, the person with pain is much more likely to make pain-control a goal.

What Family and Friends Can Do to Help

The first and most important thing that family members and friends can do to help someone deal with cancer pain is to realize this: *People with pain are the only people who know how much pain they have.* If people with pain think that others do not believe them, they can become upset and stop reporting their pain. This only makes the pain harder to control.

Family and friends can be a key to the success or failure of a pain control plan. Those family and friends involved in helping the person with cancer pain need to agree on what their role will be. Sometimes a person with cancer prefers to "go it alone." More often, the person with cancer wants someone to guide and help them, to "run interference" for them. Both the person with pain and the helper need to be clear about what is expected, wanted, and needed in the way of help and support. Here are some ideas of things family and friends can do to help a person cope with pain:

- Offer to go for a walk with them.

- Help the person devise and keep a pain diary.

- Suggest or prepare a warm shower, bath, hot water bottle, or warm washcloth to help relax their muscles and offer comfort.

- Try cool cloths or ice to soothe their pain, especially pain that comes from swelling.

- Help position the person better with pillows and soft cushions.

- Massage sore spots like the neck and shoulders.

- Help the person avoid lifting or straining.

- Encourage the person to use deep-breathing exercises.

- Provide distraction with pleasant activities.

- Help the person avoid stressful events.

- Encourage the person to expect and demand pain control.

- Watch for changes in:
  — the level of pain
  — the type of pain
  — response to pain, such as crying and being upset about feeling pain
  — ability to get up or walk
  — sleep habits
  — appetite or eating habits
  — desire to visit with friends and family

CHAPTER 2

Describing Pain

Key Points

- The person with the pain is the expert about his or her pain and pain relief.

- It is important to tell the doctor or nurse as much as possible about pain, pain relief, side effects, and other problems with pain control.

- Severe pain can be relieved.

- Severe pain should be reported right away: do not wait until your next appointment.

- Use rating scales, diaries, lists, and other methods to describe pain and pain relief.

- Describe pain in as much detail as possible.

- Tell about *all* pain, not just the pain that hurts the most.

Mary is fifty-four years old and has lung cancer. Most of the time Mary does not have pain. When Mary tries to climb stairs or walk fast, the pain is excruciating. She stops to rest a few times on her way upstairs to her bedroom. Mary wakes up each night with severe pain. When she visited the doctor, Mary was asked if she had pain. She didn't have pain right then and so she said no. She didn't tell the doctor about the pain when she climbs stairs or awakes in the night. Mary thought the pain was part of having cancer. She figured she'd have to put up with it. The doctor didn't ask any more questions about it, Mary went home, and the pain continued to interfere with her life.

Health providers used to think that all pain was alike. Pain from surgery, broken bones, arthritis, and cancer were managed in the same ways. Now we know that cancer pain is different and that relieving cancer pain is different from relieving other kinds of pain. Cancer pain can be present all the time or it can occur only at certain times. The actual cause of the pain may or may not be known. Cancer pain is different for each person. Learning as much as possible from the person with pain contributes to the best management of that person's pain.

Mary's story is common. Many people do not report pain, and doctors and nurses can forget to ask. Describing pain is not easy. Sometimes the words are hard to find; sometimes people don't really listen to the words. Some languages don't even have a word for "pain." No tests or exams show pain or describe how it feels. Pain can change from minute to minute and day to day.

A person's description of pain—where it is, when it starts, what helps to relieve it—are key to understanding cancer pain. Only the person with pain knows exactly what it is like. If a person does not describe their pain and pain relief to the doctor or nurse on a regular basis, cancer pain management is likely to fail. The person with pain is an important partner in relieving pain.

Pain Assessment

Health care providers use the word *assessment* to describe questions they ask to learn more about you and your pain. Expect your doctor or nurse to ask about your pain and pain relief at each visit: if they do not ask, and you are experiencing pain, *tell them*. Describe any changes since your last visit. The better you describe the pain, how it affects your life and activities, and what works to relieve it, the easier it will be for others to help.

Write down information about your pain and what helps to relieve it, and bring this written information with you to doctor or clinic appointments. Many people feel unsure about offering information to doctors and nurses; it is even harder to question plans for care. As clinical psychologist and cancer survivor Margaret Gosselin says, "You're sick. You're already one down. Now you have to advocate for yourself more than you ever have before in your life. There's a lot at stake here! This is important. It's about living and life!"

Questions used in a pain assessment

People express pain in different ways: some cry out, some stay still, some try to bear pain without showing it, some frown, some look sad. The way we show pain does not always tell others how bad it feels. In addition, pain that lasts a long time (chronic pain) is different from pain that lasts a short time (acute pain). With acute pain, the body reacts with changes in blood pressure and heart rate. With chronic pain, the body's reactions change: the person may not "look in pain" at all. Only the person with the pain can know and tell what the pain is like.

Pain assessment helps depict pain and pain relief in ways that everyone understands: you, the doctor, the nurse, and anyone else involved in helping you manage your pain. The information is easiest to understand if the same kind of assessment is used each time. Here are some of the questions that make up a good pain assessment. If your doctor or nurse does not ask, tell them about what is happening to you.

What is your pain like? Describe how it feels. How bad is your pain? Does it feel achy? Burning? Stabbing? Gnawing? Sharp? Dull? Or does it feel like something else?

The list below includes some of the words used to describe pain. If the pain feels like something that isn't on the list, use your own words. Be sure to tell health care providers if you use a word other than "pain" to describe what is happening. Many people use words like "hurt," "boo-boo," "discomfort," and "sore" to describe pain, which may not communicate all that you intend. Non-English words can confuse doctors or nurses who don't understand the language being used.

Some Words Used to Describe Pain

Aching	Sharp	Dull
Burning	Crushing	Pins and needles
Sore	Stabbing	Prickling
Pounding	Throbbing	Shooting
Crampy	Knot-like	Deep
On the surface	Pressing	Stretching
Tight	Pinching	Tender
Electric	Pulsing	Gnawing

Describing pain is not easy. One of the best ways to measure pain and pain relief is to use a *rating scale*. Use the list below to choose a scale that makes sense to you and is easy to use, and use it each time pain is assessed. Rating pain using a scale makes pain easier for others to understand. Ratings make pain "visible."

Scales for Rating Pain and Pain Relief

1. Numerical Scale
   Example:

   0 to 10 scale

   The person rates the pain from zero (0), meaning no pain, to ten (10), meaning the worst pain possible. Ranges such as "0 to 5" or "0 to 100" may also be used.

2. Faces Scale

   Example:
   The person points to the face that best shows the pain.

   Rating scale is recommended for persons age 3 years and older. (Reprinted by permission from Whaley, L., and D. L. Wong. *Nursing Care of Infants and Children*. 5th ed. St. Louis, Mo.: Mosby-Year Book, Inc., 1995.)

3. Words Scale
   Examples:

   1) no pain — a little pain — a lot of pain — too much pain
   2) mild — moderate — severe

   The person selects the word or words that best describe the pain.

4. Visual Analog Scale
   Example:

   |_____|
   no pain   *worst pain possible*

   The person makes a mark on the line to show where the pain is on the line.

5. Color Chart
   The person selects a color that best shows the pain. Colors are often white for "no pain" and red for "excruciating pain," with other colors in between. The person can also choose the colors that mean pain and no pain.

When using a numerical scale of 0 to 10, pain ratings of 5 or above get in the way of activities for most people. It's important to rate pain *relief* using the same scale. Write down the date, time, pain rating, relief rating, and what you did to help. Rating pain and pain relief tells how well the pain control plan is working. For example, if the pain rating stays at 9 (on a scale of 0 to 10) after taking prescribed medicine, the medicine is not working. If pain was a 9 and medicine made it drop to a 2, it shows the medicine helps.

In a words scale, "mild," "moderate," and "severe" are sometimes used to describe pain. These words mean different things to different people. Mild pain for one person may be moderate or severe pain to another. Because of this, the words must be defined: everyone involved must use the same words and know their meaning. In general, "mild pain" is a 1, 2, or 3 on a numerical scale. "Moderate pain" is a 4, 5, or 6. "Severe pain" is a 7, 8, 9, or 10.

Diaries or journals help to describe what is happening with pain and pain relief. Information can include the day, time, pain rating, what you were doing, what you tried to relieve the pain, how well it worked, any side effects, and any other comments related to pain. Keeping track of pain and pain relief helps the doctor and nurse understand what is happening when you are at home or at work and away from their care. It helps them know when to change the plan in order to control pain best.

Where does it hurt? Does the pain move from one place to another?
Tell exactly how the pain feels. Does it feel like it's on the inside of your body? Or does it seem like it is on the outside? Point to the places that hurt. Show where the pain moves if it travels from one place to another. Use a drawing of the outline of a body to show the places where it hurts. Be sure to show *all* of the places that hurt, not just the spot that hurts the most.

Do you have more than one spot where it hurts?
You may have more than one kind of pain—some caused by the cancer, some by the treatments, and some unrelated to the cancer (arthritis or a stress headache, for instance). It is important to describe each kind of pain in detail.

When does the pain happen? How long does it last? Does the pain come and go? Or is it there all the time? Is this pain new? Have you ever had this pain before? When does it begin? When does it end?
Describing pain this way helps others know more about the pain.

Does the pain keep you from doing all you want to do?
Pain may stop people from moving, walking, climbing stairs, bathing, working, playing, or getting around. Sometimes pain interferes with thinking and concentration. Pain can interfere with being close to other people. Describing how pain limits your life will help your doctor or nurse set goals with you for dealing with your pain.

Does pain interrupt your sleep? Does it change your mood? Affect your appetite?

When pain interferes with sleep, mood, or appetite, it can affect all parts of life. A first goal for treatment is to insure a good night's sleep. When you are well rested, you have more energy to try to get well, to talk with others, to enjoy life, and to do the things that are important to you. Pain can also cause you to feel grumpy or sad, especially when it lasts a long time. Pain can change the way you eat and cause you to gain or lose weight. Pain that won't go away can change the way you feel about yourself and others. Explaining how pain affects you can help others understand more about your pain and how to make it better.

What do you think causes the pain?
Many people with cancer fear that pain means the cancer is spreading or has returned. This is not always true. Pain may be caused by constipation, not moving around as much as usual, or other reasons not related to cancer. New pains can cause worry and concern. Your doctor and nurse need to know what you think is happening. Doctors and nurses will look for the cause of the pain. But even if the cause is not found, pain can be treated.

What makes the pain better? What makes it worse?
People try things to relieve pain. Some work well; others may not work at all. Sometimes pain occurs when you move a certain way. Sometimes staying in one position eases the pain. Telling your doctor or nurse about these things can help them control your pain more quickly.

What have you tried to relieve the pain?
Different kinds of pain respond to different treatment. You may have already found things that work well to relieve the pain. You may have tried relaxation, meditation, heat, cold, or mild exercise. These may all relieve some kinds of pain. If so, your doctor or nurse will want to include these actions in your treatment plan.

You also might have tried things, such as certain medicines, that did not relieve the pain. Your doctor or nurse needs to know this to avoid delays in finding just the right treatment for you.

Your doctor or nurse also needs to know all of the over-the-counter medications you take and what medicines have been prescribed for you by another doctor or nurse practitioner. Some medicines can't be taken together. Some medicines with different names contain the same chemicals and could be harmful if too much is taken.

What medicines are you taking for pain right now?
Describe all the medicines you have tried for pain in the last two or three days. Be prepared to list all other medicines as well. List the name, amount of medicine, time the medicine was taken, amount of relief, and any side effects.

How are you currently taking medications to relieve pain?
Sometimes medicines that have not worked before might be effective if they were taken in a different way. Describe exactly how and when you are taking medicines now. Your doctor or nurse needs to know if the way you are taking medicine is different from the instructions on the bottle.

Describe how long the medicine takes to work. How long does pain relief last? Does all of the pain go away after you take the medicine? Does the pain return before the next dose is due?
Answers to these questions make it easier to come up with a plan that works for your pain.

Do you have any side effects from medicines you are taking? Do you have any allergies?
Medicines for severe pain cause constipation. Dealing with constipation is an important part of the pain control plan. Expect to be asked about bowel movements at each visit. Two days is too long to go without a bowel movement when taking

most medications for severe pain. Also talk about other side effects that cause problems; most are easy to treat.

Discuss your allergies to medicines and other things. Describe how the allergy showed itself and when you first noticed it.

Do you have any worries about taking medicines for pain relief?
Many people worry about taking medicines, especially narcotics or opiates, for pain relief. They worry about addiction and other side effects. Addiction rarely occurs in people taking medicines *for the relief of cancer pain,* yet many people do not take medicines or take less than they need because of this fear. Your doctor or nurse needs to know how you feel about this. They should explain that it is not a problem. (See Chapter 3 for more information about this.) Ask questions about other worries you may have.

How much relief would allow you to get around better? What is your goal for pain relief?
You may be asked to set a goal for pain relief. The goal may be based on the ratings scale (for example, 2 on a scale of 0 to 10). Or, your goal may focus on activities you would like to carry out (walking without pain, being able to work). The aim of the treatment plan is to meet the goals you set for pain relief.

Other parts of assessment

Expect a pain assessment to include a physical exam whenever possible. Blood tests, X rays, and any other tests should be reviewed. Your past and present health history is important too. Other questions include your previous experiences with pain and pain relief and your ideas about pain and pain relief. Tell the doctor or nurse if paying for medicines is a problem. Let them know about other concerns as well. Be sure to add your own information if they haven't asked the right questions.

What Gets in the Way of Describing Pain?

There are many factors that may interfere with a complete description of pain and, therefore, its treatment. Some of these are described below.

The doctor or nurse is not comfortable treating cancer pain.
It may surprise you that many doctors and nurses learn very little about pain and pain relief in school. They mostly learn about pain on the job. Learning this way is risky. People may pick up very good information on the job, but they can also learn outdated ideas that actually interfere with pain control. Professional journals report that doctors and nurses often lack basic knowledge about cancer pain relief. Studies show that cancer pain is often undertreated, even when doctors and nurses have correct information. Pain is beginning to be a part of basic education for some doctors and nurses, but change is slow. All cancer pain can be treated. Ask to see another doctor or nurse if you think your pain is being ignored or under-treated.

The doctor or nurse doesn't ask about pain regularly. Everyone asks different questions each time. The pain assessment is not complete.
Pain should be assessed at each visit and whenever there are any changes in pain. Assessment is also key after any therapy that causes pain. Regular assessment includes using the same assessment tool and rating scale each time so that information from one visit may be compared to that from the next.

Beliefs and attitudes about pain are not correct.
Many people have pictures in their minds about how someone with "real" pain looks. The common picture is that of a person in short-term, severe pain (acute pain). Grimacing, muscle tension, crying out, and groaning are acute-pain behaviors. Acute pain is accompanied by changes in blood pressure, heart

rate, and breathing. These behaviors and changes in body functions are not always seen with long-lasting pain (chronic or persistent pain), even though the pain is severe. For someone with chronic pain, a flat, masklike expression is common. The person may have learned not to groan. There is no way to tell if a person is in pain just by looking at them. As Margo McCaffery, a well-known consultant in pain relief, says, "Pain is whatever the person in pain says it is, occurring whenever the person says it does."

People with cancer pain may not tell about their pain. Some reasons include:

- Fears and beliefs that pain cannot be treated

- Trying to be a "good patient" by not talking about pain

- Trying to be "tough" by not telling about pain

- Thinking that talking about pain will distract the doctor from treating the cancer

- Thinking pain means the cancer is getting worse

- Believing the pain will get worse if attention is paid to it

- Believing that pain is punishment and must be endured

Assessing Your Own Pain

Family members and friends can help with your assessment. If you're not up to writing the assessment, ask for help. Teach others to list your pain ratings. Bring a family member or friend along for doctor's visits. Let them help you tell others about your pain and pain relief.

Try to complete your own pain assessment using the format in the workbook in the back of this book. Use the assessment to check on your pain and pain relief between visits to the doctor. Bring the assessment with you each time you see the doctor or nurse. Use it to describe what's happening if you call on the phone. If the assessment is too hard, keep a diary about the pain. Find a way that is easiest to describe the pain and to show how much relief there is each day. Remember, the person with the pain knows the most about the pain and its relief. Share what you know with others.

CHAPTER 3

Using Medicines to Relieve Cancer Pain

Key Points

- The aim of pain control is to *prevent* the pain from returning.

- Medicines can control almost all severe cancer pain.

- Side effects from medicines should be prevented and aggressively managed.

- The pain plan may include several medicines used together.

- Medicines may need to be taken regularly whether or not you feel pain.

- Medicine for severe pain can be adjusted as needed to control pain.

- The amount of medicine you require to control your pain may be very different from the level needed by someone who has similar pain.

- Addiction is rarely a problem for people who take medicines to relieve cancer pain.

- Morphine is a good medicine for relieving many kinds of severe pain.

- Alertness and activity are often improved by treating pain with medicines.

José has pain and pressure from bowel cancer (colon cancer) all of the time. His nurse told him to take morphine pills on a regular schedule. The nurse said not to skip any doses unless he let her know, and to also take two ibuprofen tablets (Advil, Motrin IB, Nuprin) four times each day. She gave him medicine to keep his bowels regular too. She asked José to keep a diary of his pain and pain relief. He was to call if most of the pain was not gone by the next day, if the pain was worse, or if side effects were present. José was very concerned about taking "all that medicine." He especially worried about using morphine all the time. He only used the medication when his pain was really bad. He didn't call at all. Pain ruled his life.

José did not need to suffer. Many people with cancer pain have the same concerns as José. These worries get in the way of good pain control. This chapter describes medicines for cancer pain and ways to take them for the best relief. It will help you understand the pain-treatment plan.

The best way to get rid of cancer pain is to treat the cancer or to treat the cause of the pain. For example, chemotherapy or radiation can be used to reduce the size of a tumor that presses on a nerve and causes pain. When this is not possible or does not work well, medicines, alone or with other therapy, can control most forms of cancer pain.

Many kinds of medicine are used to treat cancer pain. The choice of medicine depends on the kind of pain, how severe the pain is, the cancer treatment, and other factors. Medicines can be used together to improve pain relief.

The goal of cancer pain relief is to offer the best pain relief, with the fewest side effects, in the easiest plan to follow. The easiest way to control cancer pain is to prevent it. When pain exists most of the time, taking pain medicines on a regular schedule, even when you don't feel pain, works best. Waiting until the pain really hurts makes it harder to control. It takes less medicine to treat mild to moderate pain than to treat severe pain. Preventing cancer pain, sometimes called "staying on top of the pain," lets people do the things they want without pain getting in the way.

Good pain relief does not mean the need to sacrifice alertness. Some people worry that taking as much medicine as is needed to relieve the pain means losing the ability to think clearly, to talk with family and friends, and to concentrate. When medicines are prescribed correctly and the doses adjusted to manage the pain, most people actually feel better and think more clearly than if pain persists. Pain makes it difficult to concentrate, sleep, or communicate with others. Only a very small number of people with cancer pain, whose pain is difficult to control near the end of life, will ever need to make a choice between pain relief and alertness.

Things to Know About Medicines

Each person's pain-treatment plan is unique. To create the best plan, you will need to work closely with the doctor or nurse. Tell your doctor or nurse about any medicines you take on your own. Never take someone else's medicines. Do not start or stop taking any medicines without checking with your doctor or nurse first.

The exact amount of medicine to take at one time is called the *dose.* For most pain medicines, the dose is measured in *milligrams.* A milligram is a measure of weight in the metric system and is abbreviated *mg*. One milligram is one thousandth of a gram. A gram is equal to about one twenty-eighth of an ounce. Liquid medicines are also measured in *milliliters*, or *ml*. Five milliliters is about one teaspoon. The dose of some liquid medicines is written as *milligrams per milliliter* (mg/ml).

Medicines take different amounts of time to work. Some start to work in minutes, others take several hours or even days to start to work. The time it takes for a medicine to start working is called *onset* or *onset of action*. Different medicines relieve pain for different amounts of time. *Duration* is the amount of time the effect of a medicine lasts.

These terms are important to know, especially when more than one medicine is used in the pain treatment plan. Some medicines work for two to three hours and wear off. Other medicines work for four hours or more. New kinds of long-lasting tablets last eight, twelve, or 24 hours. Skin patches can work for up to three days. When the medicine wears off, the pain may return. Doctors and nurses use the onset and duration of each medicine to decide when to schedule each dose. Taking medicine too early can cause serious side effects. Waiting too long may let the pain return. Sticking to directions is a key to success in a pain relief plan.

Many medicines have more than one name. All medicines have a *generic name*. The generic name tells what the medicine is made of. Examples of generic names are aspirin, acetaminophen, ibuprofen, morphine, and hydromorphone. Many medicines also have a *trade name* or *brand name*. The trade name is the name a company gives a medicine when they make it. For example, Tylenol, Aspirin Free Anacin, and Datril are trade names for acetaminophen. Advil, Nuprin, and Motrin IB each contain ibuprofen. M.S.I.R., Roxanol, MS Contin, Oramorph SR, and Kadian are trade names for morphine.

A brand name nonprescription medicine (or "over-the-counter" medicine) has its generic name printed somewhere on the label. Read medicine labels carefully. Compare the ingredients. It's easy to take too much of a medicine without knowing it. Ask the pharmacist for help, or check with your doctor or nurse.

Medicines Used for Cancer Pain

Medicines that decrease pain are called painkillers, or *analgesics*. These play a major role in pain relief. Analgesics do not affect the cause of the pain, but they do make pain feel less strong. Other medicines can help certain pain problems. For example, medicines used to treat depression or seizures can sometimes stop pain caused by irritation or damage to nerves. When used to relieve pain, these medicines are called *adjuvant medications* or *coanalgesics*. The term *adjuvant* refers to medicine that is "added to" or used instead of analgesics to manage pain or other symptoms. Adjuvant medications might be used to treat nausea and vomiting, sedation, and other side effects of cancer and cancer treatment.

Taking several medicines can be confusing. Be certain you understand what medicines to take, when to take them, and how to stop side effects. If you are not sure, check with your doctor or nurse.

Medicines for mild pain

Mild pain from cancer is treated with medicines called *nonnarcotics*, *nonopiates*, or *nonopioid analgesics*. Nonopiate medicines are good pain relievers. They are used alone for mild to moderate pain, or together with other medicines for severe pain. Acetaminophen (Tylenol or some other brand of nonaspirin pain reliever) or ibuprofen (Motrin IB, Advil, Nuprin, and others) work for many kinds of pain. Aspirin is a superb pain reliever but is not often used for people receiving chemotherapy or radiation therapy. Aspirin hampers blood clotting and can cause bleeding problems from even small cuts, bruises, sores; and can cause stomach, small bowel, and large bowel ulcers.

Except for acetaminophen, these medicines are in a class of medicines called *nonsteroidal anti-inflammatory drugs*, or *NSAIDs*. Some of these medicines are available without a prescription; others require a prescription. Most relieve about the same amount of pain if standard doses are used. NSAIDs' ability to relieve pain varies from person to person. Some NSAIDs relieve swelling and inflammation and reduce fever. Table 1 lists common medicines used to treat mild pain.

Table 1: Medicines Used to Treat Mild to Moderate Pain

Nonprescription Medicines	Prescription Medicines
Acetaminophen (Tylenol and others)	Choline magnesium trisalicylate (Trilisate)
Acetylsalicylic acid or aspirin	Ketorolac (Toradol)
Ibuprofen (Nuprin, Advil, Motrin)	Diflunisal (Dolobid)
Naproxen (Aleve and others)	
Ketoprofen (Orudis, Actron, and others)	

Unlike medicines used for severe pain, increasing the dose of these medicines beyond the standard dose will *not* improve pain control. In other words, there is a limit to the amount of nonopiate medicine that can be taken at one time. This limit is called the *ceiling*. Taking more than the directions on the bottle specify or your doctor or nurse suggests will not improve pain control but will cause problems. Taking too much can cause serious side effects such as bleeding, stomach upset and ulcers, kidney and liver problems, and ringing in the ears. Some products are not clearly labeled and contain aspirin, acetaminophen, or ibuprofen along with other medicines. Cold remedies and medicines for arthritis pain often contain these medicines. Be sure you know the ingredients of your medicines.

Many of these pain relievers are available in different forms. For instance, acetaminophen is available in gelcaps, caplets, and tablets. Each regular-strength tablet contains 325 mg of acetaminophen and relieves the same amount of pain. The difference is the way the pills look. For some people, gelcaps are easier to swallow. Aspirin comes in many forms, too. Buffered and enteric-coated aspirin each contain aspirin, with a special treatment that helps reduce stomach irritation.

Over-the-counter medicines can cause serious side effects. Check with your doctor or nurse before using them, and report any side effects right away.

Medicines for moderate to severe pain

The most common medicines for severe pain are *opiates* (*opioids* or *narcotic analgesics*). Table 2 lists the common medicines used to treat moderate to severe pain. These medicines all require a prescription. Unlike medicines used for mild pain, the dose of opiates or narcotic analgesics may be increased by your doctor or nurse as much as necessary to relieve the pain. In other words, with your doctor or nurse's guidance, *there is no ceiling* on the amount of these medicines

Table 2: Medicines Used to Treat Moderate to Severe Pain

All of these medications cause constipation. Be sure to ask the doctor or nurse how to prevent constipation while taking these medicines. Report any nausea, vomiting, sedation, or other symptoms as well.

Generic Name	Trade Names	Forms Available	Comments
Morphine sulfate: Short acting	MSIR Roxanol OMS Concentrate MS/L Rescudose RMS suppositories MS/S suppositories	tablets; liquids; suppositories; for injection	Each dose lasts approximately 3 to 4 hours
Morphine sulfate: Long acting	MS Contin Oramorph SR Kadian	tablets	Medicine is slowly released over time (8–12 hours for MS Contin and Oramorph SR, and 12–24 hours for Kadian).
Do not chew, crush, split, or change the pill in any way; these pills must be swallowed whole. Do not take more frequently than prescribed.			
Hydro-morphone	Dilaudid Dilaudid HP HydroStat	tablets; suppositories; for injection	Similar to short acting morphine
Oxycodone Short acting	Roxicodone	tablets; liquid; suppositories	Each dose lasts about 3–4 hours

Generic Name	Trade Names	Forms Available	Comments
Oxycodone Long acting	OxyContin	tablets	Each dose lasts about 12 hours.
Do not chew, crush, split, or change the pill in any way; these pills must be swallowed whole. Do not take more frequently than prescribed.			
Oxycodone combined with aspirin	Percodan Roxiprin	tablets	Use for severe pain is limited because of the ceiling for aspirin.
Oxycodone combined with aceta-minophen	Percocet Tylox	tablets	Use for severe pain is limited because of the ceiling for acetaminophen
Methadone	Dolophine Methadose	tablets; liquids; for injection	Needs occasional dose adjustment even if the pain remains the same. Do not skip follow-up appointments.
Fentanyl	Duragesic patch Fentanyl Oralet Sublimase Innovar	Transdermal patch; oral preparation; for injection	Patch may last up to 3 days. Oralet must dissolve in the mouth slowly.

Generic Name	Trade Names	Forms Available	Comments
Levorphanol	Levo-Dromeran	tablets; for injection	Needs occasional dose adjustment even if pain remains the same. Do not skip follow-up appointments.
Oxymorphone	Numorphan	suppositories; for injection	Use of this medicine is limited because it is not available in an oral form.
Meperidine	Demerol	tablets; liquid; for injection	Although often prescribed, **meperidine is not a good drug for cancer pain.** Use should be limited to 2–3 days. Agitation, irritability, and restlessness can occur. Report these symptoms.

that can be taken to treat severe pain. However, do not take more than is prescribed without asking your doctor or nurse, as taking too much of any medicine at once can be dangerous. But, working with your doctor or nurse, your pain can usually be relieved by slowly increasing the doses of these medications. The dose of these medicines can always be raised. *There is never a time when there is nothing to treat pain.* Meperidine (Demerol) was once a popular drug for pain control, especially after surgery. Some doctors still prescribe it today. However, meperidine is not a good medicine for cancer pain control, as taking it for more than two to three days will cause problems. As the body absorbs meperidine, the medicine gives off a by-product called normeperidine. After two to three days, normeperidine makes people anxious and restless. It also causes muscle twitches and, in high doses, can cause seizures. The Agency for Health Care Policy and Research (U.S. Department of Health and Human Services) affirms that meperidene is a poor choice for cancer pain control. In addition, some health care facilities no longer use it for surgery, especially in older people.

Side Effects from Opiates

Report any side effects from opiates to your doctor or nurse. Side effects can be managed. Do not stop taking pain medicines because of untreated side effects.

Constipation

Most medicines for severe pain, including all opiates, cause constipation. Opiate analgesics make the gut move slower. Feces, or BMs, get hard and dry. When starting medicines like morphine, hydromorphone, or fentanyl, you will need medicine to maintain regular bowel movements. If your doctor or nurse does not suggest medicine for your bowels, ask about it. It is very important to tell the doctor or nurse if your bowels have not moved for more than two days. Severe constipation causes pain, nausea, and vomiting and can be dangerous. Constipation is a potential problem as long as a person takes opiates. As doses of opiate medicines are increased, untreated constipation gets worse.

There are easy steps to take to prevent constipation, such as drinking more water and fruit juices, eating more fiber, and exercising. However, these steps are usually not enough; other medication may be needed. People sometimes stop taking medicines that can help pain because constipation is not well managed. Don't let this happen to you. Tell your doctor or nurse if your bowels are not working well. For more information about constipation, refer to page 21 in Chapter 1.

Suggestions for managing constipation:

- Take prescribed medications to prevent constipation as directed.

- Increase the amount of liquid you drink each day.

- Eat foods high in fiber, such as grains, prunes, and applesauce.

- Exercise as much as possible. Moving around helps prevent constipation.

- Maintain your usual bowel movement schedule.

- Drink warm liquids.

Nausea, vomiting, dry mouth, drowsiness, and confusion

Other serious side effects from pain medicines are rare, especially in people with cancer. If side effects occur, they are most likely to happen at the start of treatment or when doses are raised quickly. They are likely to go away after a few days. Opiates can cause nausea and vomiting, drowsiness, dry mouth, and confusion. The body builds up a tolerance to most side effects except constipation. Other medicines can help to stop these side effects. Mental status should be monitored closely, and if confusion continues it should be further assessed by the doctor and/or nurse.

Suggestions for managing nausea or vomiting:

- Take antinausea medicine for the first several days of therapy. Ask the doctor or nurse for instructions for this. Nausea and vomiting usually last 2–3 days.

- Eat small amounts of food spaced throughout the day rather than several large meals.

- Eat foods such as dry toast, crackers, oatmeal, pretzels, yogurt and sherbet.

- Drink clear liquids.

- Avoid greasy or fried foods and sweet or spicy foods.

- Use a straw for liquids and sip slowly.

- Sit up or walk around for one hour after meals.

- Avoid tight, restricting clothing.

- Get plenty of fresh air.

- Use relaxation, guided imagery, or distraction.

Suggestions for managing dry mouth:

- Drink a lot of fluids unless there is another reason to limit their intake.

- Suck on sugar-free hard candies such as peppermint or lemon.

- Take sips of fluid often, using a water bottle or thermos when away from home.

- Maintain good oral hygiene.

- Avoid commercial mouthwashes, as they contain alcohol and dry the mouth more.

- For severe dry mouth, use artificial saliva (Salivart, Orex, or Moistir). Squirt into the mouth as needed.

- Report white or red patches and any other changes inside your mouth to the doctor or nurse.

Suggestions for managing drowsiness:

- Drink beverages that contain caffeine, such as tea, coffee, or cola.

- Wait, unless drowsiness is severe, as it will usually go away within three days of starting therapy or increasing doses of medication.

- Report excessive drowsiness to the doctor or nurse. The dose of pain medicine may be adjusted, or medications can be prescribed to help.

Other side effects

Sometimes opiates can cause breathing to slow down. This is not a problem for most people taking opiates for cancer pain, and tolerance to this side effect develops quickly. Opiates can also cause bad dreams, sweating, itching, or difficulty passing water (urinating). Again, all of these side effects can be managed. Talk to your doctor or nurse.

Using Medicine to Get the Best Relief of Pain

The World Health Organization publishes the three-step *analgesic ladder* (shown in Figure 1) as a guide to using medicines to treat cancer pain. Every physician and nurse should know how to use it. In addition, the WHO offers these reminders for using medicines for cancer pain:

- Prescribe and use medicines *by mouth* (oral tablets and liquids) whenever possible.

- Schedule medicines regularly by the clock for cancer pain.

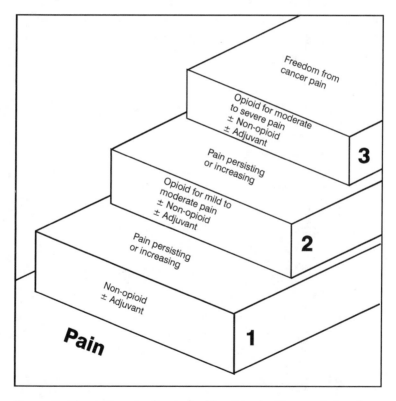

Figure 1. Three-Step Analgesic Ladder (Used with permission from World Health Organization, 1990.)

- Use the step-by-step *analgesic ladder* as a guide if pain remains or gets worse.

- Plan for each person as an *individual,* according to pain and pain relief.

- Pay *attention to detail* in assessment and treatment.

The WHO recommends analgesics for most pain. Other medicines are added for pain that does not go away with analgesics alone. Medicines can be added to treat specific problems like nausea, anxiety, or constipation. The ladder is a simple way to show how to use pain medicines systematically. As pain gets worse, move "up" the ladder. If the cause of pain goes away, move "down" the ladder. More than 90 percent of all cancer pain can be relieved using the steps shown in the ladder.

Examples of Medicines Used with the World Health Organization Analgesic Ladder

Step 1   Mild pain
Pain relievers

- acetaminophen

- aspirin

- ibuprofen

- naproxen

- ketoprofen

- choline magnesium trisalicylate

- propoxyphene

Plus, medicines to treat other symptoms such as:

- nausea

- anxiety

- pain from irritation or damage to nerves

Step 2   If pain does not go away using medicines in step one, or if pain gets worse

- Oxycodone with aspirin or acetaminophen

- Hydrocodone (Vicodin, Lortab, and others)

Step 3   If pain does not go away or if pain is severe
Doses of these medicines are gradually increased by the doctor or nurse until the pain is relieved or side effects are not manageable.

- Morphine

- Hydromorphone

- Oxycodone without aspirin or acetaminophen

- Methadone

- Fentanyl

Beyond the ladder; for pain caused by nerve irritation or damage.

- Tricyclic Antidepressants (amitriptyline, desipramine).

- Anticonvulsants (phenytoin, carbamazepine).

- Oral local anesthetics (mexiletine).

(Adapted from Agency for Health Care Policy and Research. Clinical practice guideline no. 9. *Management of Cancer Pain.* Rockville, Md.: U.S. Department of Health and Human Services, March 1994.)

When to take medicines

Using medicines on a regular twenty-four-hour schedule helps prevent pain. An around-the-clock schedule keeps the amount of medicine in the body at a steady level that controls pain and keeps pain from returning. There are fewer side effects when medicines are taken this way.

When pain only occurs during certain activities, taking pain medicine *as needed* or *p.r.n.* (Latin for *as necessary*) is okay. For instance, when pain is present *only* during a dressing change or other procedure, taking medicine just before the procedure helps. As-needed doses are also used between scheduled doses if pain returns too soon.

When pain gets better or goes away, it may be tempting to stop taking pain medicine. This lets the pain come back and starts a roller-coaster ride of some relief, then more pain. Don't stop taking your medicine even if you feel well. If the cause of pain goes away, talk to the doctor or nurse about slowly reducing the dose. Continue to assess pain and pain relief. Be prepared to stop reducing the dose if pain comes back. Stopping medicines too quickly can lead to side effects and the return of severe pain.

Some people worry that taking medicines on a regular schedule means taking too much medicine. Actually, using an around-the-clock schedule relieves pain with less medicine than would be needed if the pain were allowed to return. Using medicine for cancer pain on a regular schedule does not mean you won't be able to enjoy life. In fact, many people who take medicine for cancer pain on an around-the-clock schedule go on with work and play. They can enjoy life because pain doesn't get in the way.

The dose needed and the schedule vary for each medicine and each person. Duration and onset of action are different for each medicine too. Schedules can be confusing. Write down the scheduled time for each medicine, and record that it has been taken on the schedule. See the worksheet in the back of this book (page 139) for a sample medicine schedule.

As a rule, mild pain is treated with medicine taken every three to four hours. The need to take medicine every four hours can interfere with sleep, work, and play. If medicine is prescribed every three to four hours around the clock, set an alarm during the night to remind you to take the medicine on time. Skipping the nighttime dose will cause you to wake up with pain in the morning.

Long-acting medicines (such as MS Contin, Oramorph SR, OxyContin, and Kadian) are used for severe pain. These pills slowly release morphine or oxycodone—allowing them to act over an extended span of time. These pills must be swallowed whole. Do not crush, chew, or cut them. If the dose is not high enough, pain can return between doses, but these medicines should *never* be taken more often than every eight hours (every 12 hours for Kadian).

Pain that occurs between doses of medicine is called *breakthrough pain*. Small doses of short-acting analgesics (duration of action of three to four hours) in between long-acting doses help prevent breakthrough pain. A short-acting pain reliever like morphine (MSIR or Roxanol) can be taken every two to four hours "as needed" with a long-acting medicine. This is called a *rescue dose* for breakthrough pain, as the short-acting medicine "rescues" the person from pain until the next long-acting dose is due. Taking rescue doses more than a few times each day can be a sign that the long-acting dose needs to be higher. Keep a list of the amounts of each medicine taken, including the times and pain ratings. This information is used to adjust the plan to control pain. Fine-tuning the dose based on pain and pain relief gives the best results. Work with your health care provider to find just the right plan.

Adjusting medicines for the best relief

Raising or lowering the doses of pain medicine to get the best relief is called *titration*. Each person's pain is different, and each person responds differently to medication. Good pain relief depends on a plan that is created specifically for one person and that is adjusted as the person's pain changes. If pain gets worse, the dose may be raised or another medicine tried. If too many side effects occur, the dose may need to be lower. If other treatment stops the pain, pain medicine may not be needed at all.

Dose ranges for medicines used to treat severe pain vary according to the individual. There is no "standard dose." Some people find relief with a few milligrams of medicine. Other people need larger doses, and some may need more than several hundred milligrams. Work with your doctor or nurse to find the right dose. *The right dose is the dose that relieves pain with the fewest possible side effects.*

Assessment of pain and pain relief helps to make the right changes. Help your doctor and nurse with titration by keeping a list of the times medications are used and by rating how well each medicine works.

What Kind of Medicines Relieve Pain Best?

The best medicine depends on the kind of pain and the person with pain. There is little difference in ability to relieve pain within *groups* of medicines. In the NSAID group, two regular-strength aspirin tablets (325 mg per pill, a total of 650 mg) provide about as much pain relief as two regular-strength acetaminophen tablets (325 mg per pill, a total of 650 mg) or one ibuprofen (200 mg) tablet. Extra-strength aspirin and extra-strength acetaminophen (500 mg in each pill) are about equal in pain-relieving power. Comparing a pain-relieving dose of one medicine to another medicine's equal pain-relief dose is called *equianalgesia*.

This "equal pain-relief dose" idea also applies to medicines given in different ways. The dose of a medicine taken orally (by mouth) is higher than the equal pain-relief dose of the same medicine given by injection (shot) into the muscle (IM) or vein (IV). Pills and liquids taken orally go first to the stomach and the liver. The liver breaks down some of the medicine. About two thirds of the dose is carried out of the body in body wastes; what is left goes from the liver into the bloodstream. This medicine is then carried by the blood to the brain, where it works to decrease feelings of pain.

The same medicine given in an injection goes directly into the bloodstream to start working. For this reason, an oral dose must be about three times a dose of the same medicine given by injection to get an equal amount of pain relief. In other words, if pain is controlled with 10 mg of morphine by injection every four hours, it will take 30 mg of morphine taken orally every four hours to relieve the same amount of pain. So, whenever the way a medicine is given (called the "route of administration") is changed, the dose must be adjusted for best pain relief. If you suffer more pain after your pain-relief dose is changed from injection to oral, or suffer from side effects when it is changed from oral to injection, the dose may need adjusting and you should alert your doctor or nurse about this.

The tables below show approximate equivalent doses of medicines commonly used to treat cancer pain. Each medicine and dose will relieve approximately the same amount of pain. Compare doses when new medicines are added to your plan, especially when medicines are changed from one route of administration to another. A common error that nurses and physicians make in cancer pain management is changing from injections to pills using the same dose. For most medicines, this results in the dose being decreased by nearly two thirds. Pain will return because the dose is not high enough. Many doctors and nurses are unfamiliar with equianalgesic dosing. Share these tables with them, or tell them about the AHCPR Guidelines for Cancer Pain Management listed in the Resources section at the back of this book.

Pain medicines taken orally take about forty-five to sixty minutes to begin to bring relief. Injections into muscle (IM) start to work in about fifteen to thirty minutes. Medicines given directly into a vein (IV) start working almost immediately. More information about the ways pain medicines are given can be found in Chapter 4.

Table 3: Estimated Equal Doses of Medicines Used to Treat Mild to Moderate Pain

Medicine	Dose	Comments
Aspirin	650 mg	2 regular-strength tablets
Acetaminophen	650 mg	2 regular-strength tablets
Ibuprofen	200–400 mg	1 to 2 over-the-counter tablets
Ketoprofen	25 mg	1 over-the-counter tablet
Choline magnesium trisalicylate	500 mg	1 tablet, by prescription

Exact comparisons are not available. These doses are approximate comparisons based on prescribing information from manufacturers. Individual response may vary.

Table 4: Estimated Equal Doses of Medicines Used to Treat Moderate to Severe Pain

Medicine	Oral dose	Injected dose (IM, IV, SC)
Morphine	30 mg	10 mg
Hydromorphone	7.5 mg	1.5 mg
Hydrocodone	30 mg	not available
Oxycodone short acting long acting	30 mg 15 mg	not available not available
Methadone	20 mg	10 mg

(Adapted from Agency for Health Care Policy and Research. Clinical practice guideline no. 9. *Management of Cancer Pain.* Rockville, Md.: U.S. Department of Health and Human Services, March 1994.)

Other Medicines Used for Pain Relief

Analgesics alone don't always produce total pain relief. Pain from damage or irritation to nerves may not respond to analgesics. Some people get pain relief from antidepressant and anticonvulsant medicines. Anticonvulsants and antidepressants take several days to weeks or more to start to relieve pain. It is not yet known why these medicines work for some kinds of nerve pain, but they can help a pain plan succeed.

Medicines used to treat anxiety, sedatives, and some heart medicines can also be helpful for nerve pain. Mexiletine (Mexitil), a medicine that controls the rhythm of heartbeats, has been used for nerve injury pains when other pain treatment has failed. Codeine, capsaicin, sedatives, and antidepressants have been used for the nerve pain caused by *herpes zoster* infection, or *shingles*. Not everyone gets relief from these medicines. For others, pain might be relieved for only a short time. But sometimes the effect is long lasting. Although these medicines do not take care of pain in all cases, they do add to the number of things we can use to fight cancer pain.

Anti-inflammatory medications called *corticosteroids,* such as dexamethasone (Decadron) and prednisone, decrease swelling from cancer that presses on the spinal cord or brain. Corticosteroids may increase appetite or cause fluid retention or other side effects. Follow directions for taking corticosteroids carefully. Do not stop taking corticosteroids without letting your doctor know. With the doctor's or nurse's guidance, corticosteroids will be decreased over time until the dose is next to nothing. Then the medicine can be stopped.

Many people have pain from cancer that spreads to bone. If only one area is involved, radiation therapy can take away the pain. A fairly new treatment for bone pain involves another form of radiation. Medicine that contains tiny radioactive bits (strontium-89 or Metastron) is injected into a vein. The blood carries it to the area of bone that is damaged by the cancer. One treatment usually works within a few days (sometimes in a few hours). Relief of pain can last from a few weeks to several months. The oncologist will know if a person's bone pain can be treated with strontium. When radiation or strontium cannot be used, combining an opiate with a nonsteroidal anti-inflammatory (NSAID) often relieves the pain of cancer that has spread to bone.

Some kinds of pain respond to other medicines. Topical (applied to the skin) capsaicin (Zostrix or Capzaisin) is a cream or salve made from a chemical in chili peppers. Some people find it helpful for pain caused by irritation or damage to nerves, as in the pain from shingles. Some women find that capsaicin cream relieves the long-term pain after mastectomy. It has also been put in candies and lozenges for mouth sores. Sometimes it works; sometimes it doesn't. Capsaicin causes a burning feeling when it is first used. Some people don't like this burning and stop treatment. Others find that the burning goes away. Ask your doctor or nurse for more information.

Some people see marijuana as a useful pain reliever. Studies do not support this use. Marijuana has little physiologic effect on pain. However, ingredients in marijuana may be helpful to relieve nausea and vomiting and improve a person's sense of well-being, making pain easier to endure.

What to Know About the Medicines You Take

Be familiar with the medicines you are taking, the plan for taking them, and any potential side effects. For all medicines you take, know the following things:

- The names of the medicine (generic and trade names)
- What the medicine is for
- When to take the medicine
- How to take the medicine
- What to report to the doctor or nurse
- How to manage any side effects
- What shouldn't be taken with the medicine
- Any other precautions

Understanding prescriptions

A prescription for medicine is a legal paper that tells the pharmacist exactly what medication to give a person and the directions for taking the medicine.

A prescription has several parts:

1. The person's name, address, and date of birth. Prescriptions are given for only one person, and that person's name must be on the paper.

2. The date. Some prescriptions must be filled within a specific time or they are not valid. Ask if your prescription has a time limit. Many states limit the number of days you have to fill a prescription, especially for medications used to manage severe pain. After a certain number of days (seven in many states), the prescription cannot be filled.

3. The abbreviation Rx. This appears on all prescriptions and means "take thou." The term identifies the paper as a prescription.

4. The name of the medication. The doctor can prescribe using either the brand name or the generic name. The pharmacist *must* dispense exactly what is written unless the doctor says it is okay to substitute a similar product. With permission, the pharmacist can substitute the least expensive comparable medication. When the doctor writes the prescription using the generic name, the pharmacist can dispense the least expensive brand of that medicine.

5. The quantity. This may be written as "Dispense" or "#" (meaning "number") and tells the pharmacist how much medication to dispense.

Name: _____   Date: _____

Address: _____

_____   D.O.B.: _____

Rx

Refills: _____   May Substitute: _____

Signature: _____   DEA# _____

6. Directions for taking the medication. These follow the abbreviation *Sig,* which means "label." Directions tell exactly how and when to take the medicine.

7. A note about the number of refills that can be supplied, if any. For example: "Refill: 6 times" or "Refill: x 6." Some prescriptions for severe pain cannot be refilled; another prescription is required. Some states limit the number of pills that may be given over a certain time. These rules sometimes make pain management more difficult. If you have problems getting what your doctor or nurse prescribes, be sure to tell them right away.

8. A note or check mark to designate if a similar, less expensive product may be substituted (see 4 above).

9. The doctor's signature and address. For some medicines, the doctor's prescribing number or DEA number is also written. The DEA number is a number that allows an individual doctor or nurse to prescribe certain medicines such as opiates.

Filling Prescriptions

Have all prescriptions filled at the same pharmacy. The pharmacist should keep track of your medicines and make sure they can be taken together. Sometimes it can take more than one day to get a refill. Your local pharmacy may not carry all pain medications and may have to make a special order for them. Plan ahead for refills to avoid running out. Be sure to have enough medicine to get through a weekend or holiday. Check the number of pills left before each doctor's visit, and ask for new prescriptions before running out. Prescriptions for opiates cannot be telephoned to the pharmacy; a written prescription is needed each time.

Taking Medicines

Get directions in writing and repeat them to the doctor or nurse. Be sure you understand the directions before leaving the doctor's office. Write down the name of each medicine and what the medicine looks like. List why it is prescribed (for example, "pain control" or "bowel management"). Make a chart to help you keep track. Note the times each medicine should be taken. Cross out the time after taking the dose.

Keep medicines in the original containers. Do not mix medicines in one bottle or pillbox, as it is easy to get confused when taking many different medicines. If a new medicine does not look the same as the previous prescription, ask the pharmacist (or the nurse) about the change.

Concerns About Using Medicine for Pain Relief

Many people are concerned about taking pain medications. Fear of addiction causes many people to remain in pain. The public and even some health care providers still do not understand the difference between tolerance, physical dependence, and addiction. Doctors, nurses, pharmacists, and others who fear that a person with cancer will be addicted to pain medicine do not have current cancer pain-control information.

Concerns about addiction

Fear of becoming a "drug addict" is the most common fear about using opiate analgesics or narcotics. This concern is an old idea that even some doctors, nurses, and pharmacists still have. Yet studies show that addiction is rare in people who take opiates for control of cancer pain. Addiction is not a problem unless the person has a history of substance abuse.

Addiction is a psychological problem that causes people to take drugs *for reasons other than the relief of pain*. In other words, the person may want the medication to get "high." Experts know that addiction is *not* a problem for people with cancer pain. Studies show that less than one-tenth of one percent of all people given opioids for cancer pain become addicted. People with cancer pain use medications for pain relief. This use does not lead to addiction.

Taking opiates regularly over time does cause physical dependence and tolerance. Dependence and tolerance differ from addiction. *Physical dependence* means that if the medicine is stopped suddenly, physical withdrawal (restlessness, nasal congestion, diarrhea, muscle twitches, and other symptoms) occurs. *Tolerance* is another physical symptom that occurs when pain medicine has been used for a long period of time. The body "gets used to" the medicine, and small increases in the dose may be needed to keep the pain under control. Physical dependence and tolerance are not big problems for people with cancer pain, and they *do not* cause addiction. If the medicine has to be stopped for any reason, gradually decreasing the amount by about three fourths each day will eliminate physical dependence and tolerance.

Concerns about saving strong medicines for later

Strong analgesics like morphine used to be given only when a person was dying. Some doctors and nurses were even taught that these medications should be used only when death was close. Strong medications were "saved" until pain was terrible or death was near. Today we know that these medicines are not a last resort. Morphine and similar medicines can be given anytime pain is severe—for surgery, childbirth, chronic pain, and cancer pain. There is never a reason to "save the strong stuff until last." With your doctor's or nurse's help, the doses of these medications can be increased as much as needed to relieve most kinds of severe pain. As we said earlier, the right dose is the dose that relieves the pain with the fewest side effects.

Concerns about not being able to think clearly

People think better when pain is not a problem. In fact, a recent study shows that pain actually causes confusion in elderly people after surgery. When the dose is right, pain medicine should not cloud thinking. Some people have a little trouble for several days when a medicine is first started; most quickly adjust. People taking medicine like morphine for cancer pain can work, play, and lead active lives.

Concerns about not being able to stop taking a medicine

People in cancer pain increase and decrease doses of medicines as pain changes. When pain goes away, most people do not like the way pain medicines make them feel. Pain "uses up" the pain medicine in the body. When pain goes away, the dose of medicine is gradually lowered and stopped. Here's an example of how it works:

> *Billy is fifty-four years old and has leukemia (cancer of the blood that causes too many new white cells to form). When his white blood cell count goes too high, he has severe pain. As his blood count goes up, he starts taking morphine and gradually increases the dose until he has relief. Before his treatment for leukemia begins working, he needs what some would consider "large" doses (1000 mg of long-acting morphine) twice a day to let him continue to work. As the treatment begins to control his cancer, he works with the doctor to lower the dose of morphine until he no longer takes any. Billy then continues his life without the need for pain medicine until his cancer returns. He takes pain medicine only when he has pain. He goes for weeks and sometimes months without any medicine when his cancer is under control. He has managed his pain this way for more than five years.*

Concerns that severe pain can only be treated by injections

Almost all cancer pain can be treated by the use of tablets or pills, as long as the person can swallow, has a gut that works, and is alert. The key to relieving pain with oral medicines is to gradually raise the dose until pain is relieved. In the past, doctors and nurses did not know about increasing opioid doses to treat severe pain. The first dose was often the only dose tried before changing to a different route like shots. Now we know there is no limit to the opioid as long as the dose is increased slowly. Using pills, tablets, or liquids in doses that relieve the pain lets people get around easier. For most people, this plan is simple to follow.

Medicines given through needles, pumps, and catheters also need to be increased until pain is relieved. Medicines given this way are not more powerful than pills or liquids taken by mouth. In comparable doses, each method has the same ability to relieve pain.

There is no one right way or one right medicine to relieve the pain caused by cancer or cancer treatment. Each person's pain is different. The pain might change from day to day. There are many medicines that can be used alone to provide relief of pain. Two or more medicines can work together to get control of pain. Different routes of administration—ways to take the medicines—offer yet more approaches to success in pain control. Adding one or more of the "other ways to manage pain" described in Chapter 5 can round out the pain-relief plan. The physical and mental effects of cancer and pain must be taken into account to create a pain-relief plan that has the best chance of success.

CHAPTER 4

How Pain Medicine Is Given

Key Points

- There is a variety of ways each medicine can be given.

- The way pain medicine is given must meet the needs of the person with pain.

- When one method or route does not work well, another can be used.

Standard Routes of Administration

Pain medicines are given in a variety of ways, called *routes of administration*. The route chosen is based on your ability to take medicine. The various routes are described below and compared in Table 1.

The oral route

Taking medicine by mouth, the oral route, is by far the easiest and cheapest way to take pain medicine. Nearly all people can manage pain completely with oral medicine. Most of the opioids and nonsteroidal anti-inflammatory drugs can be given by the oral route.

Oral medicines come in pill, capsule, and liquid forms. Children might prefer liquid medicines. Tablets and capsules can be made in such a way that the medicine is released gradually in what is called *controlled-release* forms. Controlled-release medicine must be given whole in order to work the right way.

Only a very few people need to use other routes of administration during illness. People who have trouble swallowing might not be able to take pills or liquids. Digestive problems can block or impair the action of some medicines. Mouth sores or a sore throat may make it hard or painful to swallow. In addition, many people need to use more than one route to keep pain under control during the last few weeks of life. When medicine can't be taken by mouth, the rectal or transdermal route could be tried.

The rectal route

In the rectal route, medicine in a suppository is placed into the rectum. The suppository, which is made of a sugarlike substance with the medicine added in, melts from body heat and releases the medicine. Morphine, hydromorphone, and oxymorphone are pain-relieving medicines that come in suppository form.

The transdermal route

Another kind of pain medicine is put into a special patch that sticks to the skin. Over time, the medicine seeps into the skin and is absorbed by the body. So far, the only pain medicine available in this form is fentanyl (Duragesic). The transdermal route is good for people who cannot use the oral route.

The parenteral routes

Medicines that can be injected into a muscle or vein are called parenteral medicines.

Injection into the muscle, called *intramuscular* or *IM* injection, is a common way to give many medicines and vaccinations. However, it is not a good way to give pain medicines. Not only does it take longer for IM medicines to take effect, but injections are also painful and they can increase the chances of infection.

Medicines can be injected just under the skin into *subcutaneous* (SQ, Sub-Q, or SC) tissues. This route can be an alternative to IM, IV, or oral routes. The SQ route might be used when the need for pain management is expected to be limited in time or if the IV route can't be used. A continuous infusion of medicine is done using the SQ route, and the medicine is slowly absorbed through the tissues into the bloodstream.

In the *intravenous,* or *IV,* route, medicine is injected right into a vein. Used on a continual basis, this route makes for an even level of medicine in the bloodstream, provides a rapid onset of pain relief, and allows for quick dose changes. The IV route requires constant access to the veins.

In the *intraspinal* route, medicine is injected into the spinal fluid. There are temporary and permanent techniques for giving intraspinal medicine. The pain specialists will work with the patient and his or her caregivers to decide which form of intraspinal system has the best chance of success.

In the *intraventricular* route, medicine is placed in one of five small pockets inside the brain called the *ventricles.* This requires the placement of a special device (called a *subcutaneous reservoir*) just under the scalp that stores and then transfers the medicine to the ventricle. Or a pump can release medicine to the ventricle continually. The intraventricular route is fairly new and has not yet been used for a great number of people.

Patient-Controlled Analgesia

Patient-controlled analgesia (PCA) is just what the name implies: a pump system that allows the person receiving the medicine to control the amount he or she gets. PCA can be used with oral medicines, or a special pump can be used to give medicine by subcutaneous, intravenous, or intraspinal routes. A set dose is given in a constant, steady infusion. In addition, the patient can treat *breakthrough pain* on his own by using a *bolus*, or extra, dose. PCA allows the person to adjust pain medicine as needed to control pain that comes with changes in position or activity. For example, a person might use PCA to get a bit more pain medicine just before having a test or procedure that causes added pain or discomfort. PCA is safe for people in the hospital or at home. However, it should not be used by people who are confused or drowsy.

Comparison of Routes of Administration

Oral: Used when the person can swallow and digestive system function is normal

Advantages
- Easy to take
- Convenient
- Effective
- Least expensive

Drawbacks
- Must remember to take medicines on schedule
- As dose goes up, may have many pills to swallow
- Some insurance may not pay for oral medicines

Advice
- Keep track of schedule and when medicines are taken
- Check with the insurance company about coverage
- Let doctor or nurse know if the number of pills to be taken is a problem

Transdermal: *Used when a person is unable to take oral medicine and/or the person is already on opioid therapy and pain level is fairly constant*

Advantages
- Flexible dosing is possible
- One patch has a 72-hour supply

Drawbacks
- Getting to the right dose takes time
- Has a maximum dose that can be achieved
- Often requires another medicine to treat breakthrough pain
- Not suited for those needing quick dose changes
- Some people may need to change the patch every 48 hours

Advice
- Those needing higher doses can be switched to an oral, SQ, or IV route

Rectal: *(Suppository) Used when a person has nausea or vomiting, cannot swallow, or is fasting before or after surgery*

Advantages
- Simple to use
- Low cost

- Can be placed in a stoma (an abdominal opening to the bowel sometimes made during surgery for colon or rectal cancer or to help relieve a bowel obstruction)

Drawbacks
- Avoid in cases of sores in rectum or around anus
- Cannot be used when there is diarrhea
- Might be difficult for elderly or disabled person to put in place
- Some people do not like this route

Advice
- When switching from oral to rectal dose, start with same dose and increase the dose as needed

Intramuscular (IM) Injection: Used when pain control needs are expected to last only a few days—as in immediately after surgery

Advantages
- Quick to give

Drawbacks
- Difficult to predict time to work
- Is a source of pain or at least discomfort
- Injection site can allow entry of germs and cause infection
- Requires injection skills

Advice
- IM injection is rarely used in the management of cancer pain
- Consult with doctor or nurse about using a different route

Subcutaneous (SQ or SC) Injection and Infusion:
An alternative to intramuscular injection or
intravenous infusion

Advantages
- Slightly less costly than IV
- Less complex than IV
- Fewer potential problems than IV

Drawbacks
- Body's use of the medicine is not reliable
- Requires access device
- Requires skills to care for and manage equipment
- May cause skin irritation
- Increased risk of infection
- Higher cost than oral route

Advice
- Be sure that less costly and more convenient routes cannot be used
- Consult with doctor or nurse about using a different route

Intravenous (IV) Infusion: Used when person has
constant nausea and vomiting, cannot swallow, has
mouth and throat pain, is confused or has mental
status changes that prohibit swallowing medicines,
needs high doses that mean taking many tablets, or
dose changes are needed quickly and are made often

Advantages
- Less pain than IM or SQ injections
- No delay in getting the medicine
- Effective and dependable action

- Rapid onset of pain relief
- Provides constant level of pain relief

Drawbacks
- Requires intravenous access device or catheter
- Requires learning skills to manage and care for equipment
- May cause skin or vein irritation
- Increased risk of infection
- Higher cost than oral route

Advice
- Be sure that less expensive and more convenient routes cannot be used
- Consult with doctor or nurse about using other less expensive and more convenient routes

Patient Controlled Analgesia (PCA): *Usually refers to IV infusion using a pump system with the patient in control of extra doses for breakthrough pain, but can be loosely applied to any pain relief system (including oral and SQ) that the patient controls*

Advantages
- Extra dose can be given if pain returns
- Extra dose can be given before planned procedures, tests, or activities that increase pain
- Offers the patient control

Drawbacks
- Same as intravenous route

Advice
- Same as intravenous route

Intraspinal: Used when pain cannot be controlled by any other route, or when side effects like confusion or nausea limit dose increases using other routes

Advantages
- Good pain relief can be expected in most people
- Lower dose of medicine can mean fewer side effects

Drawbacks
- Requires a doctor and nurse who have a great deal of experience using this technique
- Requires exact techniques
- Requires family and professional support
- Not available in all settings
- Extremely costly

Advice
- Before this route is considered, the patient's record should show that maximum doses of opioids and coanalgesics given by other routes have failed to control pain

Intraventricular: Used when pain from head and neck cancers and tumors affecting the brachial plexus cannot be controlled by any other route

Advantages
- Might be useful when all other measures have failed to control pain

Drawbacks
- Limited experience to date
- Same as with intraspinal route

Advice
- Same as with intraspinal route

CHAPTER 5

Other Ways to Manage Pain

Key Points

- There are many things you can do on your own to help relieve cancer pain.

- Many self-care measures don't cost anything other than your time.

- Friends and family members can help with some of these methods.

- One or more of these methods can be used in conjunction with pain-relieving medicines.

- It is rare that pain is unable to be relieved by using pain-relieving medicines *and* one or more of these self-care measures.

- Only a few people need complex pain-relieving measures such as nerve blocks or surgery that cuts nerve pathways.

In addition to the use of medicines, there are many techniques that can help you feel, and actually be, more in control of pain. These pain-management ideas can be used in conjunction with medicines but are powerful even when used alone. They can help both over-the-counter and pre-scribed medicines work better. Many of these techniques of-fer the advantage of being portable: you can take them or use them anywhere, anytime. Some don't cost anything. Many don't require a doctor's prescription or even a doctor's in-volvement. They may require that you learn some new skills and be open to new ideas or ways of doing things.

Some of these techniques are called *natural, alternative, holis-tic,* or *complementary* healing methods. These include massage, imagery, relaxation, and hypnosis. Using heat or cold as ther-apy is as old as time. Music is often added to a treatment plan in the management of pain and other symptoms and seems to help many people. Exercise offers many benefits. In this chap-ter, we will review these methods and some of the basic skills needed to add these techniques to a pain control plan.

Massage

Massage, an ancient healing art, takes many forms: a simple back rub, part of a rehabilitation plan for a sprained ankle, the full-body massage given in health spas. What all kinds of massage have in common is that they involve touch—usually one person touching and caring for another. A good back rub is communication without words. It increases blood circula-tion and skin tone and relieves tension. Of course, a person can massage himself or herself—but this is not nearly so pleasing as someone else's caring touch.

Though massage therapists have had special training, most people can give a simple massage. The back is easy to reach and because of the number of muscles it involves, it is ideal for massage. *Vibration* can be added to massage by using an electric massager or vibrator. Vibration with heat can be ap-plied with an electric massager that has a heating element.

How to Give a Great Back Rub

(Adapted from Michelson, D. Giving a great back rub. *American Journal of Nursing*, July 1978.)

1. *Prepare supplies (lotion, oil, or powder—not talc).* Some people prefer perfumed oils or lotions; others like them unscented; some prefer powder. Mineral oil or vegetable oil are recommended by experts. Warm the container by holding it under hot water for a few minutes. Some people also love the feel of a warm towel or sheet.

2. *Help the person assume a comfortable position.* The usual position is lying on one's stomach or side.

3. *Find a comfortable position for yourself.* If you work in a strained position, you may hurry through the massage.

4. *Make sure your hands are warm and relaxed.*

5. *Uncover the person's hips and back.* Drape the towel or sheet over the lower hips.

6. *Place your hands on the back.* Hold your hands still for a few seconds.

7. *Begin with a light stroke to apply the oil or lotion.* Place your hands on the lower back with fingers pointing toward the person's neck. Move hands straight up the back, keeping them on the back at all times.

8. *When you reach the neck, separate your hands and bring them over the shoulder blades.*

9. *Pull your hands down along the person's sides.* Repeat this movement several times.

10. *Never put pressure directly on the spine.*

11. *Work with your thumbs on the lower back.* Use your thumbs to make short, rapid strokes away from you

toward the person's head. Work close to the spine just below the waist—first on one side and then the other.

12. *Glide your hands up to the top of the shoulders.* With both hands, knead (squeeze and release) the upper back and shoulder areas. Use medium pressure, and follow the person's response: if one stroke seems to feel really good, stay with it a bit longer.

13. *Place a hand on each hip, at nearly the level of the bed.*

14. *At the same time, move both hands up and over the back.* Rest each hand where the other hand had been, and move up the back, criss-crossing to cover the entire back.

15. *Spread the fingers on your hands, and stroke out from the middle to the upper back and shoulders.*

16. *Gently squeeze the upper arm and the muscles of the upper arm.* Repeat this several times on each arm.

17. *Place your right hand on the lower back, just to the right of the spine, with your fingers pointing toward the head.* Place your left hand on top of the right hand.

18. *Make a large circle with both hands:* follow the waist to the bed, down the side of the hip, and up to the top of the buttock. Return to the waist at the spine. (Increasing the pressure you use with this stroke might feel better.) Repeat this several times on each side, reversing your hands when you go to the left side.

19. *Keeping your hands flat, stroke the entire back lightly from the neck to the tailbone.*

20. *To end the back rub,* place your right hand lightly at the back of the person's neck and your left hand over the tailbone. Pause, and rock your left hand slightly. Remove both hands together very gently.

Therapeutic Touch

Therapeutic touch works to relieve pain after surgery, to reduce general pain, and to decrease anxiety, stress, and headaches for many people. Therapeutic touch is a new version of "laying on of hands." Touch as a healing art is mentioned in the New Testament of the Bible and has been used by women healers for centuries. This technique involves an organized system pioneered in America by Dolores Krieger, a professor of nursing at New York University. Her method assumes that illness is caused by imbalance in a person's energy system. The "therapist" becomes quiet, listening with his or her hands and "tuning in" to the person. The therapist uses his or her hands to pass over the person's body, sometimes actually touching the person, and channels energies with an intent to help or heal.

Music Therapy

Music therapy is the systematic application of music to help in the treatment of physical and psychological aspects of illness. During World War II, music was found to calm shell-shocked soldiers. Since then, music has been used in many health care settings.

The National Association for Music Therapy was founded in 1950, and there are now more than sixty American colleges and universities that offer degrees in music therapy. The music therapist combines a person's musical tastes, favorite songs and artists, and the effects of music on the person's mood to create a music therapy program for each person. Music therapists are becoming more involved in cancer care, especially in cancer care centers in large hospitals and medical centers.

The basic principles of music therapy can be used by anyone. Music can help people to relax, and it can decrease anxiety, nausea, and vomiting. People using headphones during surgery or painful tests or procedures report that listening to favorite music can help decrease pain. Music can also reduce muscle tension by masking disturbing sounds. Musical instruments that are easy to play offer even the non-musician a creative outlet. Making music with friends or family members and playing instruments like handbells, electric keyboard, and guitar offers a special experience for everyone.

In its simplest form, all that is needed for music therapy is a tape or CD player with headphones, CDs, or tapes. Choose music that matches the person's needs, moods, and taste.

Some people make their own tapes to match their moods and musical taste. To create a relaxing tape, start out with about three minutes of music to match the person's frame of mind, and add tracks that reflect a more relaxed mood. Make the tape twenty to thirty minutes in length.

Experiment with music. Listen to music at different times of the day. See what happens when you listen to various types of music. Spend about twenty minutes listening to each type of music, and then assess your responses.

The more often you use music for relaxation, the more helpful it will become. Add music to routine activities like during bathing or after a morning shower.

For more information about music therapy, contact the National Association for Music Therapy, 8455 Colesville Road, Suite 930, Silver Spring, MD 20910.

Imagery

Imagery allows people to use their imaginations to take them to a safe and comfortable place. Once they have a little practice, then through imagery, they can go to their safe place anytime. Imagery is sometimes used to help people relax. Some people incorporate imagery into their overall anticancer plan as well, using it to augment the body's ability to fight cancer. (For more information on using imagery in this way, see *Getting Well Again* by Simonton, Simonton, and Creighton, 1978.)

To find your safe place, try this exercise:

Safe Place Imagery Scripts

(Adapted from Dossey, B. M. Imagery: Awakening the inner healer. In *Holistic Nursing: A Handbook for Practice*. 2d ed. Frederick, Md.: Aspen Publishers, 1995.)

1. Let your imagination choose a place that is safe and comfortable, a place to which you can retreat at any time. This place is important and will help you survive daily stressors. Anytime you need to, let yourself go to this place in your mind.

2. Form a clear image of a pleasant outdoor scene. Use all of your senses. Smell the flowers, feel the breeze. Feel the texture of the surface under your feet. Hear all the sounds in nature, birds singing, wind blowing. See all the sights around you as you let yourself turn in a slow circle to get a full view of this special place.

3. Let a beam of light, like the rays of the sun, shine on you for comfort and healing. Allow yourself to experience the warmth and relaxation.

Distraction

Distraction—diverting attention to something else—can help a person function in spite of pain. Try any of these ideas to distract attention from pain:

- Change activities—do something else for a while

- Listen to music

- Read

- Focus on another person

- Take a walk

- Take a nap or go to bed

- Write

- Concentrate on an activity that makes you think while doing something—like playing a musical instrument or working on a craft

- Learn a new skill

The pain imagery script that follows is a distraction technique that takes about ten to twenty minutes to go through.

"Scan your body and gather any pains, aches, or other symptoms up into a ball. Begin to change its size . . . allow it to get bigger . . . just imagine how big you can make it. Now make it smaller. See how small you can make it. Is it possible to make it the size of a grain of sand? Now allow it to move slowly out of your body, moving farther away each time you exhale. Notice the experience with each exhalation as the pain moves away." (Dossey, B. M., as cited above.)

Relaxation

Relaxation methods—including quiet breathing, deep breathing, and progressive relaxation—can help a person learn coping skills that offer a sense of control and well-being. These techniques should help with pain that starts in muscles or other deep tissues. Relaxation methods work well with imagery to take attention away from the pain. Deep breathing and progressive relaxation can be done whenever a person feels a need to control stress, to relax, or to gather thoughts. A doctor, psychologist, nurse, or physical therapist can teach the following and other relaxation techniques.

Deep breathing

1. Sit in a comfortable position with feet uncrossed.

2. Put one hand on the chest and the other over the abdomen—just below the waist over the stomach.

3. Take a deep breath through the nose. This will let your abdomen expand and move your lower hand out.

4. Once your abdomen is expanded, let your chest expand and move your upper hand out.

5. Hold the air in for a few seconds.

6. Slowly exhale by making a "whooshing" sound through pursed lips.

7. Repeat several times slowly.

Progressive relaxation

1. Sit in a comfortable position.

2. Close your eyes.

3. Breathe slowly, tightening your muscles as each breath is taken in, relaxing your muscles as each breath is exhaled.

4. Start with the muscles in your feet. Work up through all the body's muscles, using the tightening-relaxing cycle.

Heat

Heat, especially moist heat, can decrease pain caused by sore muscles and muscle spasms. Heat can be applied using gel packs heated in hot water; hot water bottles; a hot, moist towel; an electric heating pad; or by a hot bath, whirlpool, or shower. A heating pad that creates its own moisture (called a *hydrocollater*) is an easy way to apply moist heat. For aching joints, wrap the joint in lightweight plastic wrap (like Saran Wrap) and tape the wrap to itself. This wrap helps retain body heat and moisture. Follow these guidelines when using heat treatments:

- ***Do not use heat over a radiation therapy treatment field, or other areas that have decreased feeling.***

- Take care not to burn or damage the skin. Use extra caution if you are diabetic.

- If a burn occurs or pain increases, stop the heat application and consult with a doctor or nurse.

- Place a soft towel or cloth between the heating pad and the skin.

- Use the heating pad for an *hour or less* at a time.

- Set the heating pad *no higher than the medium* (M) setting.

- Take care when using a heating pad if you are taking medicines that make you sleepy or if the area being treated is numb.

- Remove the heating pad before going to sleep.

- Limit the heat therapy to ten minutes at a time. Try ten minutes every one to two hours.

- Wait at least twenty-four hours before applying heat to skin that has been bruised, cut, or used for an injection or subjected to any "invasive" procedure. (Heat can increase bleeding.)

- If heat does not relieve pain or makes the pain worse, try applying cold.

Cold

Cold can reduce muscle spasms that come from joint problems or irritated nerves. Cold is the main treatment for pain caused by inflamed tissues and other swelling. Cold can stop the urge to scratch an itch. Cold can sometimes relieve pain faster and longer than heat.

Plastic-sealed gel packs provide an easy way to apply cold to a painful body part. Wrap the pack with a layer of soft cloth or towel so that it is comfortable next to the skin. Keep the pack in place by wrapping it around the body part with a 6-inch elastic bandage. They are reusable and can be kept in the refrigerator or freezer when not being used. It is also easy and inexpensive to make your own cold pack: mix one-third cup of rubbing alcohol with two-thirds cup of water in a reclosable plastic bag. Put the bag in the freezer until the mixture forms a slush. The homemade pack is ready to use. It can be refrozen and reused a number of times. An ice pack or ice cubes wrapped in a towel will work just as well. Follow these guidelines when using cold treatments:

- ***Do not use cold over any radiation therapy treatment field.***

- If the skin becomes irritated or pain increases, stop using the cold therapy and notify a doctor or nurse.

- Limit the cold therapy to ten minutes.

- Avoid use of cold over an area where circulation is poor or there is numbness.

- If the cold causes shivers, stop the treatment right away.

- Do not use cold so extreme that it causes pain.

Menthol Preparations

Menthol preparations—creams, lotions, liniments, or gels that contain menthol—are rubbed into the skin. They increase blood circulation to the area and produce a warm—or sometimes cool—feeling that is soothing and lasts for several hours. Common brands include Ben-Gay, Tiger Balm, Icy Hot, Heet, Vicks Vaporub, and Mineral Ice.

Before applying a menthol product to a large skin surface, do a skin test. Rub a small amount in a one-inch circle in the area of pain to test whether the menthol irritates the skin or causes any other problem. Wait at least thirty minutes. If there is no sign of redness or swelling, rub more product into the area. Using a menthol product right after a warm shower or wrapping the area with plastic wrap after the product is applied can increase the time the menthol effect lasts. Some menthol products contain an ingredient similar to aspirin. If you have been advised not to take aspirin, check with the doctor or nurse before using a menthol product. *Do not use a heating pad over a menthol product: it can cause a burn.*

Biofeedback

Biofeedback methods use special machines to help people control some body functions such as heart rate, blood pressure, and muscle tension. Tension in muscles, joints, and connective tissue is a normal reaction to pain. The tension can actually increase sensitivity to pain. Reducing tension through biofeedback is often used along with other pain-relief measures.

In biofeedback, sound and vision provide feedback on body (or biological) functions. That's where the term *biofeedback* comes from. The biofeedback machine gives immediate visual and aural information on whether muscles are becoming more or less tense. This helps people learn to relax their muscles. During the biofeedback session, electrical leads are attached to the skin surface. The person learns to detect negative changes in the body and to reverse them before they cause more pain. In this way, biofeedback can help a person feel more in control.

The doctor, nurse, social worker, physical therapist, or other health care professional can help locate a colleague who is skilled in teaching and using biofeedback. For biofeedback to work, the person using it has to practice. Though biofeedback does not work for everyone, it is one more weapon in the fight against cancer-related pain.

Acupressure and Acupuncture

Acupressure is an Asian healing technique that includes the Japanese form, called *shiatsu,* and *reflexology.* Acupressure can be useful in pain and stress management and can be performed by a layperson. Research shows that endorphins, the body's natural morphine-like substances, are released when acu-points are pressed, warmed, or needled. According to acupressure theory, acu-points, or tsubos, are points of decreased electrical resistance that follow the body's energy paths. These paths form the meridian system. Pressure is placed on points or meridians to release blocked energy, or chi. Stimulation of the tsubos, the meridian, or a portion of one or more meridians can improve energy flow and affect organs that are distant from the area being stimulated. During acupressure, acu-points are held with a firm, gentle pressure for a few minutes or until tension goes away.

Acupuncture evolved from acupressure. In acupuncture, fine needles are inserted just under the skin to relieve pain and open energy flow. Some practitioners wire the needles to stimulate nerve endings electrically (called *electroacupuncture*) which, in theory, causes increased endorphin output. Acupuncture is performed by licensed practitioners.

Exercise

People with cancer are often advised to rest or take it easy. Long periods of bedrest and decreased activity, however, can result in a loss of function and energy. People who exercise have less tension, anxiety, depression, and fatigue. Exercise can also help control nausea that is related to chemotherapy or radiation.

Exercise programs should be started *only* after a medical checkup, including a review of other health factors like heart function, blood pressure, and problems with knees, ankles, or back. Symptoms that might prevent a person from taking on an exercise program—and suggest the need for a more in-depth medical checkup—include the following:

- an irregular or resting pulse of more than 100 beats per minute

- frequent leg pains or cramps

- chest pain

- rapid onset of nausea during exercise

- dizziness, blurred vision, or feeling faint

- bone, back, or neck pain that is new

- fever

- shortness of breath

For people with access to a swimming pool or beach, swimming or just moving around in water is a good, relaxing, and even comforting form of exercise. Check with the doctor or nurse before swimming, especially if you have a vascular access device in place, skin injuries, or other things that put you at risk for infection.

Walking is easy and good exercise. Shoes should be designed for walking or jogging with a soft midsole and skid-proof outer sole. They should lace up (or close with Velcro fasteners) and have smooth, soft insides that will not cause blisters or sores. Wear loose-fitting clothes when walking. In winter, a hat or hood will prevent heat loss.

Humor

Laughter and humor are important for coping with pain and healing. People who enjoy humor also have a better morale and a greater sense of well-being. Humor increases immune system activity that seems to help prevent infections. It helps relieve anger, anxiety, and tension. Humor and laughter improve breathing and heart and blood vessel function; muscle and bone structure and function; hormone production; and immune function. A treatment program at the City of Hope Medical Center in Duarte, California, encouraged people to use audio tapes of comedians such as Will Rogers, Jack Benny, and Erma Bombeck.

Animals and Pet Therapy

Animal lovers already know, on some level, that the bond between people and animals is helpful. More and more, this no-
tion is being explored as a basis for legitimate therapy. This
story appeared in a nursing journal:

> *Eight-year-old Jack was hospitalized for over 3 months. He had*
> *several procedures and surgeries. He was in a great deal of pain*
> *and was often frightened, which made the pain worse. A gentle*
> *English Setter therapy dog named Perri began visiting him. Dur-*
> *ing these visits, Jack was relaxed and playful. He stopped request-*
> *ing pain medications during Perri's visits, and this calm feeling*
> *eventually extended to other times.* (Barba, B. E. The positive
> influence of animals: Animal-assisted therapy in acute
> care. *Clinical Nurse Specialist* 9(4):199–202, 1995.)

Studies show that animals improve the well-being of elderly,
disabled, and hospitalized people. Physical benefits of being
with animals include lower blood pressure and heart rate and
decreased muscle tenseness. Animals can help reduce stress
and anxiety and invite people to socialize. Pets make us
laugh, decrease our loneliness, make us feel safe, and encourage us to exercise. Animals can also raise our self-esteem:
they offer unconditional acceptance, and our physical appear-
ance and manner of speech are not important to them. More
health care facilities—including hospices and oncology and
intensive care units—are including pet therapy in their list of
services. An animal can make a clinical setting feel more like
home. Whether the pet has fins, feathers, or fur, many people
say they just feel better with an animal present.

For more information about animal-assisted therapy, contact the Delta Society, P.O. Box 1080, Renton, WA 98057.

Hypnosis

Hypnosis is a trance that offers a state of intense awareness and focused concentration. Although hypnosis requires the help of a skilled therapist, it can change how pain is perceived, decrease anxiety, and increase coping skills. It has been found helpful for children who are going through painful procedures such as lumbar puncture, bone marrow aspiration, and biopsy. Adults have found self-hypnosis (also called *autohypnosis*) using audiotapes to be useful in managing some types of pain. Autohypnosis offers a sense of control over pain and other symptoms. There have been only a few studies to assess the value of hypnosis in managing cancer pain, and it is not possible to predict who it might help.

TENS (Neuroaugmentation)

TENS (transcutaneous electric nerve stimulation) is a method of bringing on pain relief by applying electrical stimulation to the skin. Mild electric currents are applied to areas of the skin by a small power pack connected to electrodes. The buzzing, tingling, or tapping sensations seem to interfere with pain sensations. The current can be adjusted up or down so that the sensation is pleasant and also relieves pain. TENS has not yet been used extensively for cancer pain, but a few studies have reported good results. A doctor, nurse, or physical therapist can help decide whether TENS might help relieve your pain. The doctor prescribes the use of TENS, and the physical therapist applies it, instructs in its correct use, and monitors its effects.

Other Approaches

Nerve blocks

A nerve block is an option for someone with severe pain that has not been controlled by other, simpler means. A local anesthetic, steroid (like cortisone), or alcohol is injected into or around a nerve, and the nerve is no longer able to transmit pain. Local anesthetics and cortisone injections offer pain relief that lasts from several days to a few weeks; phenol or alcohol offer longer relief of pain. A nerve block with phenol or alcohol can cause permanent muscle paralysis and loss of all feeling in the affected area. The success of a nerve block depends on the skill of the doctor performing the procedure.

Surgery

When pain is still severe after all other pain therapy fails, there are operations that can be used to relieve pain. In general, this type of surgery cuts the nerve's pathways—the pathways that relay the feeling of pain to the brain. A neurosurgeon (a doctor who specializes in surgery on nerves and of the nervous system) may be able to cut a nerve close to the spinal cord, a procedure called a *rhizotomy*. Or bundles of nerves in the spinal cord itself can be cut in what is called a *cordotomy*.

This type of surgery is done only after serious study. Once cut, these nerves cannot be put back together. When the nerves that transmit pain are destroyed, pressure and temperature can no longer be felt. Function and feeling that was normally controlled by that nerve or group of nerves is lost forever. In addition, the person is more prone to injury because he or she no longer has the protection offered by natural reflexes.

Pituitary ablation

Pain that is widespread and has not been controlled by other methods might respond to destruction of the pituitary, a pea-size gland at the base of the brain. The pituitary controls hormone production. Since some tumors and pain syndromes relate to hormones, destroying the pituitary can limit hormones' effects, thus decreasing pain levels. A chemical is injected directly into the pituitary, destroying it. Pain relief occurs quickly. Clearly, this technique has serious complications and side effects.

In our own lives, each of us discovers things that just plain make us feel better. We all have pleasant memories that can give us comfort. There might be techniques or things that your parents did when you were a child to "make the hurt go away." Try them now. Or you might find your own remedy, your own method, for relieving pain. You can share your success to help others in pain. A good thing to remember is that when you have pain, you are not alone. There are lots of methods to try, and there is always help. *Cancer doesn't have to hurt.*

CHAPTER 6

Finding and Getting the Most from Cancer Pain Treatment

Key Points

- A team approach is usually best for effective pain management.

- The person with pain is the head of the pain-management team.

- Asking questions is never a bother.

- Telling about problems and concerns is crucial for successful pain management.

- Preparing for a visit to the doctor or nurse ensures a more effective visit.

- There is never a time when nothing more can be done to relieve pain.

My daughter was being seen by a cancer doctor, eye specialist, endocrinologist, urologist, anesthesiologist, social worker, nurse, and psychologist, and no one was treating her pain. Worse yet, everyone gave me a different story about what to do. I didn't want to make a scene or cause trouble. I was afraid speaking up would compromise my daughter's care, but I had to do something. I started writing a lot of things about her pain in a notebook. I took the book with me every time we saw someone for care. I checked off questions when they were answered. I asked everyone to write instructions in the book too. I brought along a pamphlet about treating cancer pain. Some of my family thought I was going too far. Some of the people caring for my daughter were not very happy. But when I was confused, I took out the book. I asked each person caring for my daughter to read the instructions from others and write their own. Even they were surprised at how confusing the messages were.

It was really hard to tell those people they were not doing a good job with my daughter's pain. I worried a lot about what they would think. I was scared they'd give up on us. If it wasn't for her pain, I don't think I could have done it. I had to do something. But the greatest thing happened! After a while, everyone started asking for the book and wanted to know what was going on. They talked and put one person in charge of coordinating all the plans so everyone knew what was happening. And the best thing of all is that her pain got better. She could do some of the things a kid should do, even if she has cancer. Then they started using my idea of "the book" for other people in pain. It really made me feel good to know I was helping others too. It was worth all the sleep I lost worrying about talking to them! And most important, it helped relieve my daughter's pain.

Finding Effective Cancer Pain Relief

People with cancer often have several health care providers, including the family doctor, cancer specialists, nurses, therapists, and others. Some people get treatment in large cancer centers. About 80 percent of all people with cancer find help from doctors in their own communities.

It would be ideal if all health care providers knew the latest information about cancer pain control. Sadly, this is not the case. Recent studies show that cancer pain is often undertreated, even by some cancer specialists. Not everyone knows what to do for cancer pain. Some do not understand that cancer pain *can* be relieved. No single doctor, nurse, or pharmacist can know everything about all health care problems. Finding a health care provider can be a challenge. Sometimes insurance plans limit choice. Sometimes it's travel, time, or knowing where to go that gets in the way.

Asking questions can help you find someone who is interested in your pain control and who knows what to do. Below is a list of questions that can help you learn about a provider's interest and skill in managing cancer-related pain. Add your own questions to the list.

- How do you feel about cancer pain?

- How do you treat cancer pain?

- Is pain management important here?

- Who is part of the team?

- What happens if my pain is not relieved with the usual treatment?

- Is severe pain considered an emergency here?

- Who do I call after hours?

- How much am I involved in the plan?

- Is an assessment tool used? Which one?

- Will I receive directions in writing?

- Who will teach me about the plan?

- How is the plan communicated to others?

- Do you follow the Agency for Health Care Policy and Research (AHCPR) guidelines?

- Who can help when you are away?

- What happens if my pain does not go away?

The Cancer Pain Team: Who's on It and Who's in Charge

Pain management works best when everyone involved in your care knows about the plan. *Team approach* and *coordinated care* are phrases that describe health care providers working together to plan and provide care. A team approach makes use of the skills and talents of each person involved in care. If you get care from more than one doctor or nurse, be sure they talk to one another about your pain management. When a team approach is not used, there is room for confusion. People may get different plans from each health care provider. One plan might work against another. Teamwork gets the best results.

The person with pain is the head of any team for pain control. Only the person with pain knows when pain is relieved and what plan is easiest to follow. Doctors, nurses, pharmacists, social workers, psychologists, family, and others can be members of the pain team. Each member has a defined role to play. The doctor is often the one who prescribes pain medicine. A physical therapist might work to stretch tight muscles that can make pain worse. The nurse helps assess pain, teaches about the plan, and works with the person in pain to be sure the plan is right. A psychologist can teach relaxation exercises or help deal with stress and anxiety. Separate visits to each team member can help them get to know you better and understand your pain problem. When all of these people plan and work together, chances for better pain relief increase.

Many things help improve pain control. Pain relief is best if team members each offer ideas about what will work best and all talk together with you to come up with a plan. A good plan includes information about how to relieve the pain, who to call, when to call, and what to report. Good pain management identifies severe pain as an emergency, with help available twenty-four hours a day.

Each person's pain is unique. Pain specialists agree that the person with pain is the expert. While this is true, each member of the team must also "own" the pain. Each person giving care must feel responsible and understand the plan, and each must be responsible for listening carefully to a person's reports about pain. A responsible provider returns phone calls promptly and makes careful adjustments to the plan as needed.

Most cancer pain can be controlled by any doctor, nurse, or other health care provider in the United States who has good information about cancer pain management. Accurate information is easy to find. The Agency for Health Care Policy and Research is a division of the United States Department of Health and Human Services. The AHCPR publishes a resource for professionals that gives clinical practice guidelines for cancer pain control and that costs just a few dollars. The Patient Guide from AHCPR is free. To order a free AHCPR Patient Guide, call 1-800-4-CANCER. Other suggestions are listed in the resources section at the end of this book.

A team approach can be informal or formal. Doctors, nurses, and others who regularly talk about a person's pain control can be a team. However, when doctors and nurses cannot relieve pain using the information they know, a referral to pain specialists can help. Some health care facilities offer pain teams, consultants, pain clinics, or pain services. These services are not always needed for cancer pain control. But when pain is not controlled, pain specialists may be able to help.

Sizing Up Pain Services, Clinics, and Programs

Pain programs, clinics, and services are springing up every-
where. Many are connected with health care facilities. Some
are private practices. Most pain programs treat chronic pain
like back pain, headache, and other noncancer pain. Some
treat all kinds of pain, including cancer pain. Some specialize
only in cancer pain and symptom management. Others offer
only one kind of therapy for pain such as acupuncture or
nerve blocks.

Members of the pain team may be doctors who specialize
in cancer (oncologists), the nervous system (neurosurgeons or
neurologists), or anesthesia (anesthesiologists). Other kinds of
providers who specialize in pain include nurses, pharmacists,
psychologists, chiropractors, and physical therapists. Other
providers, who have taken a special interest in pain but don't
formally specialize in one of these areas, might also play a role
in cancer pain management.

A good pain service or clinic for cancer pain offers help
from more than one kind of health care provider; this is called
multidisciplinary or *interdisciplinary* care. Using knowledge and
skills from more than one specialty improves options for pain
control. First and foremost, look for a program that includes
you in devising a plan for your care. Select a program that
treats cancer pain most of the time and in which you will be
seen by more than one kind of provider. Be sure each provider
takes part in planning for your pain relief. In general, be cau-
tious about a service that offers only one form of treatment or
involves only one provider. Pain is complex, and good pain
relief involves using a variety of resources. In addition, the
program should designate one person to be responsible for coordinating your care.

Be certain there is a way to report if the pain is better or
worse. Ask about follow-up visits. Referral to a "single service"

pain clinic is all right when another provider is coordinating the pain-control plan. For example, when medication does not relieve pain caused by pancreatic cancer, a nerve block can improve comfort for some people, and a referral to a neurosurgeon or anesthesiologist who can do this technique is proper.

Below is a list of what you might look for or expect to find in a good pain program, service, or clinic.

- People who treat cancer pain regularly

- The use of a team approach that includes help from a variety of professionals

- The inclusion of the person with pain in planning

- Twenty-four-hour coverage for problems

- Prompt return of phone calls

- Regular contact to check on pain relief

- The inclusion of a thorough physical exam

- Questions about the effects of pain on your life

- Questions about how you are dealing with pain

- A review of tests done previously and the order of new tests if needed

- The use of a standard assessment

- The designation of one person to coordinate your care

More About Team Members: Who Does What

Pain team members come from many health care disciplines. Each has a separate role and job to do, but each member and each job is part of an organized system that works to find the best way to manage your pain.

Doctors diagnose and treat medical problems and plan medical care. They are authorized to prescribe medicines. Usually a person has a regular doctor (primary physician) and is referred to other specialists as needed. In small hospitals or community hospitals, the roles can be quite clearly defined. There is likely to be a doctor, a nurse, a pharmacist, and perhaps a social worker or psychologist. Things get more complicated in large medical centers and teaching hospitals. Many facilities provide experience for students in training to be doctors. Students and doctors have different titles depending on their education. The *attending physician* has completed training and is fully qualified to plan medical care. He or she is responsible for medical students and doctors in training. *Fellows* are doctors who are continuing training in a specific area such as cancer care or pain control. When a fellow completes training, he or she is an attending physician and is considered a specialist. *Residents* are doctors who have completed medical school and are in their second, third, or fourth year of experience after medical school. *Interns* are doctors in their first year after medical school. *Medical students* are studying to be doctors. Sometimes it's tiring and confusing to see so many different doctors. If their messages are different or unclear, ask the attending physician. This is the doctor who's in charge of your medical care.

Nurses are educated to give nursing care and to carry out the medical plan. In hospitals, *registered nurses* coordinate care, administer treatments and medications, teach, and counsel. They explain what is happening and how to take care of yourself. Nurses are often coordinators for pain clinics and services. Nurses, sometimes with the help of social workers, work with patients and families to plan for your care at home. This is called *discharge planning. Registered professional nurses* (RNs) are licensed by each state. *Licensed practical nurses* (LPNs) and *licensed vocational nurses* (LVNs) work under the direction of registered nurses. *Advanced practice nurses* in cancer care and pain management (nurse practitioners and clinical nurse specialists) have additional education (usually a master's degree) beyond basic nursing education. In some states, advanced practice nurses can prescribe medicine and be primary care providers.

Pharmacists often join the team too. Pharmacists help decide which medicine fits into a plan best, fill prescriptions, teach about medicines, and give advice about over-the-counter medications.

Social workers and psychologists are sometimes team members. They help people cope with the effects of pain. Some teach ways such as relaxation, imagery, and self-hypnosis to control pain. Medical social workers help people and their families deal with illness. Social workers help locate medical equipment, home care support, transportation, financial assistance, and other resources.

Physical therapists help with strength and movement. They design exercises that increase comfort. In addition to the people listed above, other people join the team as their services and talents are needed for pain control.

Your role on the team

Remember, the person with pain is a team member. In fact, the person with pain is the *head* of the team! Be sure to discuss your needs and wishes about pain control. Let the team know if parts of the plan don't make sense to you. Keep them informed about your pain and pain relief. Be an active team member!

Making the Most of Your Appointment

Visits to the doctor can be very helpful or very confusing. For best results, take an active role in the visit. Describe your pain, attempts at pain relief, what works and what doesn't work, and any side effects and other problems you have had with the plan. Share assessment information openly. Don't feel like you are taking too much time, and don't feel rushed. Write down information so you can review it later. Plan ahead to make the most of the visit.

Communication

Research shows that people do better and receive more complete care when they feel they talk well with the doctor. Communication is a two-way process in which each person must both talk and listen.

Good communicators ask questions that cannot be answered with a simple yes or no. The best questions need answers that give information and detail. For example, the question "How are you today?" can be answered with one word like "okay," "fine," or "terrible." No other detail is needed. But "Tell me what's happening with your pain today" invites a more informative response.

Good communicators use words that are easy to understand. Sometimes health care workers forget that most people don't understand medical terms. Remind others to use words you know when they explain things. Ask for an explanation of every word you do not understand. All medical terms can be explained using nonmedical words. Sometimes drawings or pictures help. Keep asking until it is clear. There is no such thing as a silly or stupid question. Once an explanation makes sense, you may want to ask for it in writing so you can review it later on.

Insist on being treated like an individual rather than a number or a disease. Describe your work and family. Explain what works best for you and how you want to be treated. Let others know how much information you want, and tell them how you learn new things best. Do you learn best from pictures? From being shown? From reading? Also let others know your goals. What do you want to happen as a result of this visit? What do you want to happen as a result of the care you will get? Find a provider who is a good match for you and your needs. If your situation offers little choice, at least let the provider you have know your needs. If you don't explain what you need, you probably won't get it.

Expect full attention to your problems. Do not let others rush your visits. Insist on a private place for important discussions; the hallway or reception desk is not the place to talk about personal things. Do not leave until your questions are answered fully and you have had the chance to share the information you wish.

Many people feel nervous or anxious when they visit the doctor, which may make it hard to remember what happened during the visit. Even though you listen carefully, you may not hear all that is said. Do what is necessary to understand. Ask the doctor or nurse to repeat things. Take notes. Better yet, bring a family member or friend along to listen and take notes. Tell the doctor or nurse someone is with you and that you want them to be present during the visit.

Consider tape-recording important discussions. Let the doctor or nurse know you want to record the session. The tape recording lets you listen to the discussion at a later time as often as you need to understand. Sharing the tape with loved ones lets them hear the same message. Some people videotape important sessions. As being in front of a camera is uncomfortable for many people, discuss this option with your health care provider ahead of time.

Doctors and nurses are people too. They have bad days and good days. Tell them when your plan needs a change, and let them know when their advice helps. Sharing respect will build trust.

On one hand then, you need to demand a certain level of care and attention to your needs. On the other hand, as a team member, you have responsibilities too. You can address both these goals by getting yourself organized and ready for each visit to the doctor. The list below suggests ways to prepare for your visit.

- Prepare before you go.

- Write questions ahead of time and bring them with you.

- Consider tape-recording important discussions.

- Bring someone with you to help listen.

- Speak frankly with the doctor or nurse.

- Work toward mutual trust and respect.

- Report what is really happening—all of it!

- Take notes during the visit.

- Repeat what you think you have heard.

- Don't leave until all your questions are answered.

- Insist on privacy.

- Tell how much information you want to have.

- Ask for definitions of medical terms.

- Ask what other help is available.

- Ask what you can do to help.

- Take an active role in your care.

- Do not let others make you feel rushed.

- Understand the plan and follow-up before leaving.

When to Call the Doctor

Calling the doctor is not easy for many people. Preparing ahead helps make the call more useful. Call if instructions are unclear or if you are confused about what was said. Do not wait until the next appointment if pain is not relieved. Plan ahead to have enough medicine over weekends and holidays, and call ahead for refills. In addition, call your doctor about cancer pain control for any of these reasons:

- If pain is not relieved

- If pain gets worse

- If there is new pain

- If the medicine wears off before the next dose is due

- If you experience any side effects that are problems

- If you are too sleepy to keep your eyes open or can't stay awake in a conversation

- If you haven't had a bowel movement in two days while taking opiates

- If the pain is constant, in one spot, and getting stronger

- If the pain causes you to cry out, stay still, or double over

- If there is new redness, swelling, or pus

- If you have hives, itches, or rashes

- If you are seeing things that are not there

- If you experience uncontrolled muscle movements (twitches or jerks)

- If you are feeling depressed, hopeless, or helpless

What should I say when I call about pain?

Before calling the doctor or nurse about pain, make a list of any problems and all the medicines you are now taking. List the exact times you have been taking each pain medicine for the last two days, including the time of your last dose. Write down anything else you have tried to relieve the pain and how it worked. Rate the pain now and right after you take the medicine. Give a pain rating for the best the pain has been and the worst it has been in the last two days. Have the name and phone number of your pharmacy ready. Place the bottles of medicine within easy reach when you call. List any side effects from medicine or from pain.

When you talk to the doctor or nurse, give your name and describe what is happening. For example: *"This is Jim Murphy. You are treating me for cancer, and I am having pain. I'm taking the medicine you prescribed (say the name and dose if you can, exactly as it says on the label) and my pain is an 8 on a scale of 0 to 10. Since yesterday, the pain has not been lower than a 7. I've tried using heat and relaxation with no change. I'm having trouble sleeping. My bowels are working fine. What changes do I need to make?"*

Before calling the doctor, think about each question in the following checklist:

- How long has the pain been a problem?

- Where is the pain? Is there more than one spot?

- How severe is the pain? Rate the pain and the pain relief.

- Describe the pain in words.

- Does the pain burn or feel like an electric shock?

- Is there numbness or tingling?

- What activities does the pain interfere with?

- For each medicine you are taking:
  — What is its name?
  — How much time goes by between doses?
  — How many pills are taken at one time?
  — Exactly how much medicine have you taken in the last two days?
  — How long does the medicine take to work?
  — Rate how well it works.
  — How much relief does the medicine give?
  — How long does the relief last?
  — Does the pain come back before the next dose?

- What else relieves the pain?

(Adapted from *Home Care Guide for Cancer*. Philadelphia: American College of Physicians, 1994.)

What If the Doctor Says Nothing Else Can Be Done?

Remember, cancer pain *can* be relieved. There is always something that can be done to increase comfort. Disagreeing with or confronting a doctor or nurse is not easy, but if pain control is not good, your comfort and quality of life are at risk. Bring information about pain and pain relief with you for clinic and office visits. For example, bring a copy of the

AHCPR *Management of Cancer Pain: Adults. Clinical Practice Guideline Quick Reference for Clinicians* listed in the Resource section at the back of this book. Ask the doctor or nurse to review and discuss it with you. Bring your own copy of the AHCPR *Patient Guide.* Make pain relief an important goal by being as informed as possible.

Many people find it easier to get the help they need by asking a family member or friend to join in the visit and help advocate for their needs. Discuss your needs and concerns before the visit so you both are aware of your goals. A family member or friend can help with difficult discussions, offer support, and ask some of the hard questions while you listen.

Doctors and nurses do not like to see people in pain. It goes against the purpose of their work. But poor pain relief is often the result of a lack of information, a lack of time, and placing a low priority on pain relief. If pain remains and the doctor says nothing more can be done, ask for another opinion. Ask to see someone who specializes in cancer pain relief. It is okay to request a second opinion. Experts agree that if a health care provider is uncomfortable about referring for a second opinion, that's all the more reason to *get* a second opinion. No one health care worker can know everything there is to know about all health problems. Remember, what is at stake is the quality of your life.

CHAPTER 7

Paying for Pain Treatment

Key Points

- Good pain control is part of good cancer care.
- Cost should not limit access to pain-controlling medicines.
- There are many kinds of funds to help pay for pain-relieving medicines, techniques, and care.

Good pain control is part of good cancer care. Good cancer care happens in all kinds of settings—small community hospitals, rural doctors' offices and clinics, large medical centers.

Access to doctors and nurses who know how to take care of cancer pain, access to prescription medications, and, sometimes, access to special supplies are the keys to good pain relief. In the United States, access to care, prescription medicines, and supplies are based on a person's ability to pay for them. Payment can come from our own pockets, private insurance, or one of the government's health insurance plans (Medicare or Medicaid). People with low incomes or on fixed incomes are sometimes forced to choose between spending money on food and other necessities or buying pain medicines.

It is crucial that the person with cancer or a family member or friend knows the ropes about how to pay for pain medicine. Prescription medicines are the most important part of cancer pain management. Insurance coverage affects access to these medicines: if the person with pain can't afford to pay for it and the insurance won't cover it, then the person is likely to go without the prescribed medicine. In dealing with prescriptions for pain, it is crucial to know what to expect from insurance: What will it pay for and what will it not pay for? What questions need to be asked and answered? What options are available?

Medicare

Medicare covers some, but not all, health care costs for people over sixty-five and people who have been disabled for at least two years. Most Americans over sixty-five pay for prescription medicines themselves. For the most part, Medicare does not pay for prescriptions unless the person takes the medicine while in the hospital or during an office visit. Once a person leaves the hospital and prescriptions are filled on an "outpatient" basis, the person must pay for them. The need for prescription coverage is one reason people with Medicare purchase additional Medicare insurance policies, called Medigap or Medicare supplemental insurance.

Medicare does pay for prescriptions as part of its hospice benefit. The Medicare hospice benefit allows a person who is terminally ill (thought to have less than six months to live) to receive care, including outpatient prescriptions, from a Medicare-certified hospice. Other hospice benefits include home care, respite care, and acute inpatient care.

Medicaid

Medicaid is the public health and prescription medicine insurance program for low-income people who are elderly, blind, disabled, or have dependent children. Medicaid programs are run by the individual states, and they differ slightly from state to state. The income level that qualifies a person or family for help is set by the state. Most state programs cover medicines that are given by injection in a doctor's office, by home health care nurses, and in extended care facilities. Outpatient pain medicines are covered in most Medicaid programs.

Some state Medicaid programs limit the number of times a prescription can be refilled or the amount of medicine that can be given with each prescription. Some states limit a person to a small number of prescriptions each month.

Medicare and Medicaid benefits can, in some cases, be combined to help people who qualify. A nurse or social worker can provide information about Medicaid. Application for Medicaid starts in the local or county office of the Department of Social Services.

Private Insurance

Private insurance policies vary in their payment for prescriptions. Some states allow insurance companies to sell "bare bones" policies that will probably not cover outpatient prescriptions. Private insurance companies vary in their willingness to pay for the services of clinical nurse specialists, nurse practitioners, physical therapists, psychologists, chiropractors, and other types of health care providers who could be involved in a pain treatment program. Table 1 will help you to evaluate medical insurance and benefits according to common policy features.

Table 1   Medical Insurance Benefits Compared

Feature	Rating		
	Very good	Fair	Poor
Lifetime maximum	Unlimited or $1,000,000	$500,000	Below $500,000
Specific illnesses excluded	None		Yes, e.g. heart disease, cancer, and AIDS
Days of hospital coverage per year	365	120	21
Calendar-year deductible	$100–$200	$300–$1,000	$5,000 or more
Pre-existing condition exclusion	None	1–3 months	12 months
Coverage when traveling out of home area	Yes	Anywhere in USA but not abroad	No
Prescription drugs	$3 copayment per prescription	Yes, but subject to deductible and coinsurance	Not covered
Definition of prescription drugs	Recommended in the medical literature	Allows drugs to be used even if the FDA has not specifically approved its use for this purpose	Allows use of drugs strictly according to FDA guidelines

Feature	Rating		
	Very good	Fair	Poor
Allows or permits and pays for consults with specialists *not* in the insurance/ HMO plan	90–100%	70%	0–50%
Outpatient psychotherapy	Unlimited	30 visits at $50 each	Not covered
Home care services reimbursed	Skilled care, custodial care, homemaker services	Skilled and custodial care only	Skilled care only
Hospice care	Unlimited	Limited to 6 months	Not covered

(Adapted from Cancer Care, Inc., materials. For the complete checklist, contact Cancer Care, 1180 Avenue of the Americas, New York, NY 10036-3602 or call 212-221-3300.)

Health Maintenance Organizations

Health maintenance organizations provide comprehensive health care by member doctors and referral to outside specialists. Most people enrolled in HMOs have coverage for prescriptions, including pain medicines. If prescription coverage is not part of a basic HMO plan, this benefit may be able to be purchased at an extra cost. Some HMOs require a deductible or copayment for prescriptions. Some HMOs control the type, brand, and amount of medicine that can be prescribed. In many cases, a special technique or medicine might require approval (called *preauthorization*) before treatment can be started. Limits on home care visits and access to other services and providers are often conditions of an HMO contract.

Other Sources of Funds for Pain Treatment

The ability to pay for pain-relieving medicines and treatments cannot be allowed to limit access to pain relief. Everyone has the right to expect and to receive good pain control. Sometimes, confusing insurance plans or government policies and regulations can make finding and paying for treatment of cancer pain, well, a pain! The good news is that there are many sources of help available. Every person can find comfort and relief from pain.

Not everyone has private insurance, and many people without it do not qualify for Medicare or Medicaid. Some private insurance policies do not cover the cost of the medicines prescribed for pain.

There is help. Some companies that make pain medicines have programs to supply them (sometimes free, sometimes at a lower cost) to doctors whose patients cannot afford to buy them. Because of prescription regulations, the doctor must contact the company—it is illegal for a company to give these medicines unless a doctor requests them. Ask your nurse, doctor, or social worker for help. The Pharmaceutical Research Manufacturers of America has compiled a directory that lists companies with these programs. You can get a copy of the *Directory of Prescription Drug Patient Assistance Programs* by calling the Pharmaceutical Research and Manufacturers of America's toll-free number 800-PMA-INFO, or 800-762-4636. In the Washington, DC area, call 202-393-5200. Leave your name and address with the answering service, and the list will be mailed to you within a week.

The American Cancer Society (ACS) can help people with limited incomes find help in getting pain medicines. Some state divisions of the ACS have funds to help low-income people pay for pain medicines.

Some hospitals, clinics, and other health care agencies have funding to help pay for the costs of medicines for people with cancer. Many agencies, even some in small cities and towns, have special funds set aside to help pay for the costs of care and medicines. Social workers often know about funds available in that hospital or clinic and can check whether a person qualifies for assistance.

CHAPTER 8

Special Needs

Key Points

- Every person, regardless of age or personal history, deserves good pain control.

- Good pain control is possible for everyone.

- Pain means different things to different people.

- People vary in how they react to pain.

- The basic guidelines for cancer pain control are the same for all people.

- Some people need special care and techniques to control pain.

Children, older people, people with health problems aside from their cancer, and people with emotional problems or mental illness have special needs when it comes to cancer and pain treatment. Substance abuse—either drugs or alcohol—makes for a special challenge in the management of cancer pain. Additionally, each person's life experiences must be taken into account in the care of cancer pain. In this chapter, we will look at special needs and how to address them.

Children and Cancer Pain

Children are not always offered good pain relief. Just as with adults, there are many mistaken ideas about children and pain that get in the way of good pain relief. These include the beliefs that children, and especially babies, don't feel pain; that kids have a high risk of addiction to opioids; that opioids cause breathing problems for children; and that children don't remember pain. Some people believe children can't tell you where they hurt and that they get over pain more quickly than adults do. *These ideas are myths!* Children of all ages *do* feel pain. They do not have a higher risk of addiction than adults do. (And an adult's risk of addiction when being treated with ample doses of analgesic opioids is less than 1%.) There is little risk of breathing problems when the opioid dose is based on the patient's weight. For children and infants, pain can even be life-threatening. When a baby or child cries for long periods of time, the oxygen supply to the brain and tissues can drop to dangerous levels. Special studies prove that children can indeed tell us where they hurt.

While children may recover from pain within the same time frame as adults, they have less control over the situation and know less about what is happening to them. A child's experience can actually be more frightening and thus requires special attention. And, as with adults, it is simply unethical to withhold pain relief from a child or baby. Infants also can and should be treated for pain.

The safe care of children in pain requires special knowledge, attention, and skill on the part of health care providers. Some children will have pain that is hard to control. If this is the case, specialists in children's pain should be brought in to help develop a pain care plan. Using everything that is known about pain management will bring a better quality of life to children of all ages who have cancer.

Managing pain from cancer treatment

Cancer pain in children can't always be compared to cancer pain in adults. Pain from treatments and procedures is more common in children. (In adults, pain more often relates to the cancer itself.) Partly, this contrast relates to the kinds of cancers that affect babies and children. And though the treatment of most childhood cancers results in a rapid decrease in pain, the ongoing nature of treatment and check-ups means that the child will go through painful procedures throughout the course of the illness.

Assessing pain in children requires different methods from those that work for adults. Special assessment tools have been designed for use with children: some use colors that the child can relate to pain; others have simple drawings of faces that reflect how the child is feeling. Like adults, children can tell us where they hurt—perhaps by pointing to areas of their bodies, indicating spots on a doll or teddy bear, or pointing to the painful spots on a drawing of a body.

Making sure that the very first procedure is not frightful will help a child cope with future painful procedures. The child and his or her family should know what to expect from any procedure. To the maximum extent, pain and anxiety have to be managed. The treatment room should be as pleasant as possible.

An anesthetic cream called EMLA can help reduce the pain of some needle sticks used to draw blood or to access a port, bone marrow puncture site, or lumbar puncture site. The cream is applied to the place where the needle is to be inserted and is covered by a special dressing (for at least sixty minutes) that helps the cream be absorbed into the skin. The area will be numb for around four hours. EMLA is not used for needle stick sites used to give some kinds of chemotherapy, because its effect makes it hard to ensure that the chemotherapy is going into the vein.

A pain-control technique used especially for children is *conscious sedation*. The American Academy of Pediatrics defines conscious sedation as "a minimally depressed level of consciousness that retains the patient's ability to maintain a patent airway independently and continuously, and respond appropriately to physical stimulation and/or verbal command." In other words, the child is drowsy but can breathe well on his own and follow commands. Conscious sedation is done by combining several medicines to achieve the desired effect. The medicines are given by mouth, or by IV if the child has a long-term catheter in place. The goal is to avoid the pain of needle sticks and the anxiety caused by the procedure.

Many experts recommend the use of conscious sedation when a child has his or her first lumbar puncture (also called spinal tap) or bone marrow aspiration as a way to lower the child's distress over procedures that will be repeated often. When a child is especially nervous or anxious, or where a painful procedure can be expected to take longer than about fifteen minutes, conscious sedation might be used to control the child's pain and anxiety. At one respected children's hospital, about one of every eight children getting spinal taps is thought to need conscious sedation. In this hospital, a spinal tap usually takes less than fifteen minutes. For this short period of time, simpler methods of pain control are more common.

Using medicines and other pain-control techniques

The amount of medicine used and the way medicines are given are often different for children than for adults. The correct dose of medicine is based on the child's weight and the type of pain the child has. Most children can take medicines by mouth, though some may not want to: these children quickly become suspicious of things they are given to eat or drink. Maybe the control over what they take is the last bit of control they have. In this situation, there is good reason to use the IV route of administration. Most medicines come in a liquid form for oral use, or they can be mixed in a liquid by a pharmacist. Medicines can be crushed (unless the medicine is in a time-release form) and put in a small amount of liquid or soft food. When this is not possible, children can get their medicines in the same ways as adults (see Chapter 4, "How Pain Medicine Is Given," p. 75). Children as young as five, for example, have been taught to use patient-controlled analgesia (PCA) pumps.

Pediatric nurses tell us that children, particularly teenagers, have heard the "Just Say No to Drugs" message. So even though they have pain, they may be afraid of taking drugs. It can be helpful for a trusted adult or possibly another child who has dealt with pain to discuss the difference between the bad drugs they hear about and the good aspects of the effects that pain-relieving medicines can offer.

Along with medicines, some of the other ways to manage pain described in Chapter 5 can also work for infants and children. Infants find comfort in breastfeeding, sucking on a pacifier, and being rocked. Infants and toddlers respond to distraction, music, and the comforting presence of a parent. Children can be massaged and stroked. Heat and cold can be applied. Young children and teenagers can use imagery, relaxation, biofeedback, music, art, hypnosis, and self-hypnosis to help relieve pain.

The Elderly and Cancer Pain

The elderly need and deserve good pain assessment and management. However, for several reasons, older people are likely to be undertreated for their cancer pain. Some people think that elderly people are not as sensitive to pain, that they tolerate pain better than younger people, or that pain is a natural part of aging. Older people are often given weaker medicines because the doctor or nurse wrongly assumes that the elderly cannot tolerate opioids. And some older people are confused and cannot tell others about their pain.

In truth, older people may have more pain than younger people. Older people with cancer often have other illnesses and more than one source of pain. Many older people take several medicines that don't work well together, causing adverse side effects and more pain. Older people often have problems with their eyesight and hearing, which makes communication more difficult. People who are forgetful may not be able to recall details of the pain they have—when it starts, what makes it worse, what makes it feel better. Their reports of pain may change often and quickly. As a result, older people need to have their pain levels checked more frequently than people who are younger.

As we age, our body functions change. These normal changes and those that result from illnesses must be factored in when prescribing medicines. Elderly people generally have less water in their body, less muscle mass, and more body fat. Some medicines depend on body water, muscle, fat, and protein to work in the right way. In addition, most medicines pass through the liver and kidneys. As liver and kidney functions change with age, the way the body uses, responds to, and rids itself of medicines also changes.

These changes mean that the elderly are more sensitive to the effects of certain medicines and less sensitive to other medicines. Elderly people are more sensitive to NSAIDs, opioids, and some of the other medicines used as "adjuvant" medicines to treat cancer pain. This does not mean that these medicines should not be used for older people, but the people using these medicines and their caregivers must be careful and watchful. Table 1 lists some of the concerns associated with medicines used in the treatment of the elderly.

A successful pain-control plan will take advantage of all that is known about pain-relieving medicines and all that is known about the physical and emotional changes that accompany aging. A thoughtful plan of care can provide good pain relief and allow an elderly person the quality of life that is deserved.

Table 1: Pain Medicines and the Older Person

Medicine	Concerns	Advice
NSAIDs	Increased risk of stomach irritation, kidney problems, constipation, and headache	* Ask about ways to protect your stomach when taking these medicines. * Report any signs of upset stomach. * Expect to have occasional blood tests to monitor kidney function. If problems occur, the dose may need to be decreased by the doctor or nurse.
Opioids	These medicines work quicker and longer in older people because their kidney and liver functions are slower, and the body does not get rid of the medicines as quickly.	Report confusion or sedation, especially when using long-acting opioids.
Local anesthetics (lidocaine or opioids)	May result in mental status changes, retention of urine, constipation, and blocked colon.	Monitor your passing of water, bowel movements, and any change in mental status. Report changes to a nurse or doctor.
Anti-depressants	May cause dizziness (especially when getting out of bed) and clumsiness, putting the person at risk of falling.	Notify the doctor or nurse if this happens. Sit for a few moments before standing when getting out of bed. Use a cane, walking stick, or walker, or ask for someone's support.

Emotional and Psychological Issues

Almost half of all people with cancer, especially those in pain, experience emotional and psychological problems in coping with their illness. Problems that require the help of a psychiatrist occur fairly often, most commonly during the terminal stage of illness. A person's mood and personality can be changed by severe pain; relief of pain may make the problems go away. After the pain is controlled, the mental status should be assessed again. If the problem is still there, it can be managed.

Feelings of hopelessness, worthlessness, guilt, and suicide are symptoms of depression. A person who is depressed can benefit from the help of a psychiatrist, psychologist, or mental health nurse who understands the emotional turmoil that often accompanies cancer. Depression in a person with cancer can be treated as depression is usually treated—with psychotherapy, some self-care techniques, and antidepressant medicines. Special care needs to be taken when prescribing medicines for depression when medicines for pain are also being taken. Opioids given with some of the medicines used to treat depression can cause severe reactions.

Even though very few people with cancer commit suicide, pain that is not controlled increases the risk of suicide. Fear of uncontrolled pain is a major factor in requests to doctors for help in dying, called *assisted suicide* or *euthanasia*. On the other hand, many people who consider suicide change their minds when pain is finally controlled. Quick relief of pain and other distressing symptoms is a priority for people at risk of suicide.

Delirium is common in people with late-stage cancer. In delirium, the person can be alert one minute and drowsy the next. His thinking, memory, attention, and behavior might change from normal to abnormal and back again. Delirium can be caused by the direct effect of cancer on the brain. It can also be caused by the effects of medicines, infection, imbalance of the body's fluids and chemicals, or failure of a vital organ or system. Some of the medicines that people with cancer take can bring on delirium. Opioid analgesics can cause confusion, especially in the elderly and people near the end of life. All possible causes need to be explored before the right treatment can be started. Some delirium can be reversed, but when several organs fail, delirium can mark the last day or two of life.

Substance Abuse

The treatment of cancer pain affecting people who have a history of substance abuse, or those who are current abusers, usually requires the help of an expert in both substance abuse and cancer pain. The challenges presented by this group of people, however, do not exclude them from good cancer care or good pain control. The doctor and nurse will have to consider the substance abuse in planning for pain relief but must still adhere to the general guidelines for managing cancer pain. During the assessment phase, it is common practice to place the substance abuser into one of three categories: (1) addicts who are abusing drugs at the time of their treatment for cancer pain; (2) former addicts who no longer abuse drugs; and (3) addicts in methadone maintenance programs.

People who are currently abusing drugs are likely to have developed some *tolerance* to the opioid used for pain. They will need higher starting doses and more frequent doses than people who are not addicted. Many active substance abusers will need treatment for other mental health problems. People who have abused drugs in the past or who are in a methadone program are likely to have developed opioid tolerance. They will probably need higher opioid doses given in shorter intervals.

Except in a few cases, the choice of pain-relieving medicines is not really different for people with a history of drug abuse. Some kinds of pain-relieving medicines *should not* be used for people who are now abusing opioids. These medicines block the effect of opioids, resulting in withdrawal and an increase of pain. These medicines are pentazocine (Talwin), butorphanol tartrate (Stadol), dezocine (Dalgan), and nalbuphine hydrochloride (Nubain).

Cultural Differences

Bill and Malcolm are both twenty-six years old. Malcolm is a successful bank vice president. Bill plays professional baseball. Both had similar knee injuries from sports, and both had surgery yesterday. After surgery, Malcolm was very quiet. He did not show his pain. In his family, groaning was not a good thing to do. In fact, all his life he was taught to keep pain inside. He didn't move much because the pain was so bad. He tried to think of other things to take his mind off the pain. Sometimes he prayed. Everyone assumed Malcolm did not have pain. Bill groaned, moaned, and had a pained expression on his face. He was worried this would end his baseball career. The pain scared him very much. It was a reminder that he might be out of work. His family wanted to know about his pain. Every time someone came to see him, he told them how much he hurt and how terrible the surgery was. They expected him to cry out if it hurt. Everyone felt bad for Bill and tried to make his pain go away.

Bill and Malcolm had similar pain but expressed it very differently. Malcolm endured his pain, while Bill expressed his pain openly and often. Why did Bill and Malcolm act so differently? What influences the way people react to pain?

Pain is a personal experience. Pain is complex. It involves a physical feeling of hurt and a personal reaction to that hurt. Many things influence the way a person reacts to pain and pain relief.

People learn to express pain early in life. Families and friends teach us how to express pain. Some people are taught to hold pain in; others learn to speak out or cry. Cultural beliefs and family ideas about pain behaviors relate to age, sex, occupation, the kind of problem causing pain, the amount of pain, and the length of time pain should be endured. We learn how to respond to pain, who to tell about pain, what methods can be used to relieve it, and what kind of pain needs attention. Religious and cultural beliefs and practices play strong roles in teaching us how to express pain. For some, pain is necessary and honorable and must be endured. For others, pain is bad and without purpose. Some cultures view showing pain as shameful or weak.

The source of pain also influences how a person reacts to pain. Pain from running a marathon leaves runners tired but fulfilled, especially if they have run well. The pain is quickly dismissed. Pain that threatens health is harder to endure. Cancer pain has a more negative meaning. Pain from cancer causes worry, and worry causes more pain. Some people view cancer pain as a sign of failure. Others feel it is a necessary part of having cancer.

A person's experience with pain and pain relief affects how pain is viewed. When a person knows from experience that pain can be relieved, it is less scary. A person who has had terrible, unrelieved pain will be far more frightened. Being frightened, anxious, or depressed makes pain worse.

There is no right or wrong way to react to pain. Let others know your needs and wishes, especially if they differ from usual. Below is a list of things to consider about your beliefs and values concerning pain. You may want to share this information with your doctor and nurse.

- What are your beliefs about pain?

- How do you show pain? What words do you use?

- What does pain mean to you?

- How do you normally treat and cope with pain?

- Is it okay to have someone else present during your physical exams?

- How do you gather information?

- How much information do you want?

- Who makes decisions about your health?

- What are you willing to try?

- Are there things that must be included in a pain plan for it to work for you (customs, behaviors, values, food preferences, etc.)?

- Are there things that you do not want to use for pain relief (food taboos, specific medicines, other treatments, etc.)?

- Is there anyone else who needs to be part of your plan?

- Do you have other beliefs, rituals, or taboos related to pain?

Health providers in the United States do not always consider ethnic, cultural, or religious beliefs as part of health care. For some, alternative forms of healing, other healers, and nontraditional health practices are just not acceptable. This lack of sensitivity to cultural issues may lead to poor communication, poor treatment, and increased pain and suffering. Finding a health care provider who is willing to consider other health beliefs and practices is a challenge, but for many people, a plan that allows for individual health beliefs and practices has a better chance to succeed.

Records for Keeping Track of Your Care

Keeping records of your pain control plan makes it easier for others to tell if the plan is working. Records can also help prevent confusion about medicine schedules. Choose the records that make sense for your care. Not all records will be right for everyone. If none of these records help, consider keeping a journal, or diary, or notes about pain and pain relief. Doctors and nurses use this information to determine changes in the plan to bring relief.

Make copies of these records, and use them to keep track of pain and pain relief. Bring them to your visits to the doctor or nurse. Ask them to write new medications and therapies on the record.

The *List of Medicines and Side Effects* form simply lists all of the medicines in the pain control plan. You can also include other medicines that you are taking. Some people like to make another list each day showing the exact times to take the medicines. Cross out the time on the list after taking the medicine. This list can help you keep track when many medicines are prescribed.

The *Pain and Pain Relief Record* is a way to keep track of pain and pain relief and to report side effects from medicines. There is also room to write about any other methods you tried to relieve the pain. This form helps to show the doctor or nurse if the plan is relieving pain and tells them about unmanaged side effects.

Describing Pain is an assessment form that can help you tell others about the pain. It takes a little time to complete, but this assessment can help the doctor or nurse to better understand your pain.

Some Tools to Describe Pain shows several different ways to rate pain and pain relief. Any of the scales will work, as long as you use the same scale each time pain is rated.

List of Medicines for Pain and Side Effects

Name of Medicine	Dose or amount	What it is for	What it looks like	When to take it	Side effects to report

(For a full-size chart to photocopy, see pullout. If your book contains no pullout, call Hunter House Publishers at 1-800-266-5592.)

Instructions:

1. List each medicine and the amount to be taken each time.

2. Write down what it is for (such as pain, constipation, or nausea).

3. Describe what it looks like (such as purple pill or clear liquid).

4. Write the exact time of day you plan to take it (such as 8 a.m. & 8 p.m. for twice a day; or 8 a.m., 12 noon, 4 p.m., 8 p.m.,12 midnight, and 4 a.m. for every four hours).

5. List any side effects you should report (such as no bowel movements or a queazy stomach).

Pain and Pain Relief Record

Date	Time	Pain rating	Medicine used & amount	Other things I tried	Relief rating	Side effects or other problem	Comments

(Adapted from Agency for Healthy Care Policy and Research. *Managing Cancer Pain: Patient Guide.* Rockville, Md.: U.S. Department of Health and Human Services, March 1994.)

(For a full-size chart to photocopy, see pullout. If your book contains no pullout, call Hunter House Publishers at 1-800-266-5592.)

Instructions:

1. *Pain rating*: Choose a rating scale from Chapter 2.

2. *Relief rating*: Rate the amount of relief one hour after taking pain medicine using the same scale.

3. *Other things I tried*: List anything you tried to make the pain better (such as heat, cold, relaxation, or staying still).

4. *Side effects or other problems*: List any problems, and keep track of your bowel movements.

5. *Comments*: Write anything else you wish to share (such as the location of the pain or what you were doing when it occurred).

Assessment Form for Describing Pain

1. What does the pain feel like?

2. When did it start?

3. Is it always there, or does it come and go?

4. How bad is it? (Use a rating scale from Chapter 2.)

5. Where does it hurt? (Mark the body drawing to show where it hurts.)

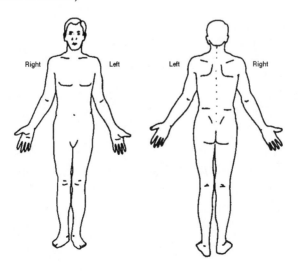

6. Does the pain move from one place to another? Where does it travel?

7. Is there more than one kind of pain? Describe each separately.

8. When do you have pain? (All the time? Only at night? Other times?)

9. How long does the pain last?

10. Is this pain new?

11. What does the pain prevent you from doing?

12. Does the pain interrupt your sleep? Do you wake up in the night or in the morning with pain?

13. Does the pain change your mood?

14. Does the pain affect your appetite?

15. What do you think is causing this pain?

16. What makes it ease off or get better?

17. What makes it worse?

18. What have you already tried to help the pain? What did you do and how did it work?

19. What medicines are you taking now for the pain?

20. How well do the medicines work to take away the pain?

21. Describe any side effects you are having from the pain.

22. Do you have other problems that make the pain harder to take?

23. Do you have concerns about the medicines you are taking? If so, what are they?

24. Do you have other concerns about the pain plan?

25. How much relief would let you get around better?

26. What is your goal for relief?

Some Tools to Describe Pain

Pick one tool that makes sense to you. Use the tool to show pain and how much relief you get from medicine and other things to manage pain.

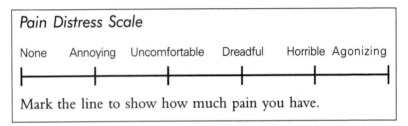

Pain Distress Scale

None   Annoying   Uncomfortable   Dreadful   Horrible   Agonizing

Mark the line to show how much pain you have.

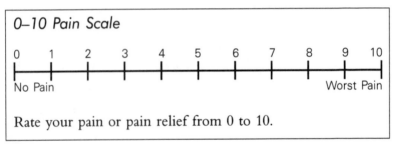

0–10 Pain Scale

0   1   2   3   4   5   6   7   8   9   10
No Pain   Worst Pain

Rate your pain or pain relief from 0 to 10.

Faces Scale

Rating scale is recommended for persons age 3 years and older.

Point to the face that best shows how you feel.

(Reprinted by permission from Whaley, L., and D. L. Wong. *Nursing Care of Infants and Children.* 5th ed. St. Louis, Mo.: Mosby-Year Book, Inc., 1995.)

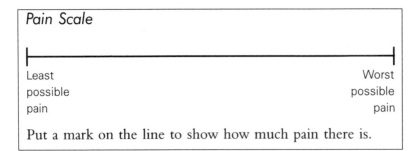

Pain Scale

Least
possible
pain

Worst
possible
pain

Put a mark on the line to show how much pain there is.

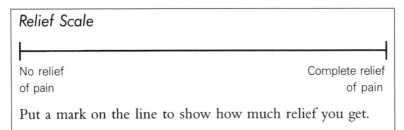

Relief Scale

No relief
of pain

Complete relief
of pain

Put a mark on the line to show how much relief you get.

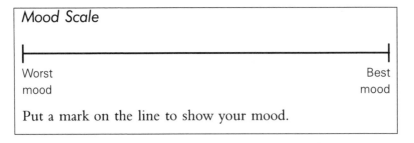

Mood Scale

Worst
mood

Best
mood

Put a mark on the line to show your mood.

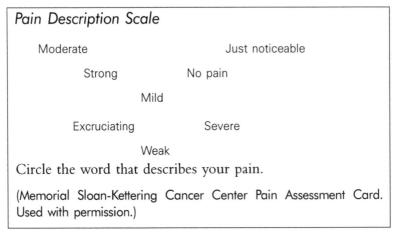

Pain Description Scale

Moderate   Just noticeable

Strong   No pain

Mild

Excruciating   Severe

Weak

Circle the word that describes your pain.

(Memorial Sloan-Kettering Cancer Center Pain Assessment Card. Used with permission.)

Resources for Cancer Pain Management

Cancer resources are easy to find. The National Cancer Institute, the American Cancer Society, the Leukemia Society of America, and cancer centers throughout the United States publish free or lowcost information about nearly all aspects of cancer and cancer treatment. This list highlights resources for information about cancer pain. You can also find excellent books, audiotapes, and videotapes about relaxation, massage, acupressure, acupuncture, guided imagery, and other self-care methods to reduce pain in local libraries and bookstores.

Publications by the Agency for Health Care Policy & Research (AHCPR)

The Agency for Health Care Policy and Research is part of the U.S. Public Health Service, and a division of the U.S. Government's Department of Health and Human Services. AHCPR convenes panels of experts to write clinical practice guidelines for common health conditions in the U.S., and guidelines for the management of acute pain and cancer pain are among the AHCPR's publications.

AHCPR Clearinghouse
P.O. Box 8547
Silver Spring, MD 20907
Tel.: 800-358-9295

Acute pain management

Acute Pain Management: Operative or Medical Procedures and Trauma. Clinical Practice Guideline. February 1992. AHCPR Publication No. 92-0032. (145 pages; several dollars)

Acute Pain Management in Adults: Operative Procedures. Quick Reference Guide for Clinicians. 1992. AHCPR Publication No. 92-0019. (23 pages; free)

Acute Pain Management in Infants, Children & Adolescents: Operative and Medical Procedures. Quick Reference Guide for Clinicians. 1992. AHCPR Publication No. 92-0020. (22 pages; free)

Pain Control After Surgery: A Patient's Guide. February 1992. AHCPR Publication No. 92-0021. (13 pages; free)

Management of Cancer Pain

These publications are available from AHCPR and from the National Cancer Institute's Office of Cancer Communications at 1-800-4-CANCER.

Management of Cancer Pain. Clinical Practice Guideline. March 1994. AHCPR Publication No. 94-0592. (257 pages; several dollars)

Management of Cancer Pain: Adults. Clinical Practice Guideline Quick Reference for Clinicians. March 1994. AHCPR Publication No. 94-0593. (29 pages; free)

Managing Cancer Pain. Patient Guide. March 1994. AHCPR Publication No. 94-0595 (in Spanish, Publication No. 94-0596). (21 pages; free)

Resources from The Wisconsin Cancer Pain Initiative

The Wisconsin Cancer Pain Initiative was the first statewide organization in the United States to focus its efforts totally on improving cancer pain control in Wisconsin. The Initiative was part of a pilot project of the World Health Organization and has become the model for almost all of the fifty states to establish individual state organizations. The Wisconsin Initiative has established a national Resource Center that provides information, materials, and support throughout the U.S. In addition to the resources listed below, displays for professionals and the public are available.

Wisconsin Cancer Pain Initiative
Cancer Pain Resource Center
Medical Science Center, Room 3671
1300 University Avenue
Madison, WI 53706
Tel.: 608-265-4013   Fax: 608-265-4014
e-mail: wcpi@facstaff.wisc.edu

Children's Cancer Pain Can Be Relieved. 1989. For parents of children with cancer. (50¢ plus postage & handling.)

Communicating About Cancer Pain. Thirty minute videotape. ($14.95 plus shipping & handling. Call 800-757-4354 to order.)

Eight Facts Everyone Should Know About Cancer Pain. (2-page pamphlet; 25¢)

Jeff Asks About Cancer Pain. 1990. For teenagers. (50¢ plus postage & handling.)

Is Cancer Pain Inevitable? Thirty minute videotape. ($14.95 plus shipping & handling.)

Resources from the American Cancer Society and the National Cancer Institute

American Cancer Society
1599 Clifton Road
Atlanta, GA 30329-4251
800-ACS-2345   (800-227-2345)

Or contact your local unit or state division of the American Cancer Society, or the National Cancer Institute's Office of Cancer Communications at 800-4-CANCER (800-422-6237).

Cancer Information Service
National Cancer Institute
Office of Cancer Communications
Center Drive, Building 31, Room 10A10
Bethesda, MD 20892-2580

Questions and Answers About Cancer Pain Control: A Guide for People with Cancer and Their Families. 1992. American Cancer Society/National Cancer Institute. Publication No. 92-200M-4518. (76 pages; free)

Get Relief from Cancer Pain. 1994. American Cancer Society/National Cancer Institute. ACS Publication No. 94-4517 PS. (6-page pamphlet; free)

Other Books and Pamphlets

A Bill of Rights for People with Cancer Pain. Available from Cancer Care, Inc., 1180 Avenue of the Americas, New York, NY 10036. Tel.: 212-221-3300.

Cancer Pain Education Program: A Comprehensive Approach to Pain Management in the Home. Two audiotapes, instructions for sixteen nondrug interventions for pain relief, self-care logs, and a booklet, *Managing Cancer Pain at Home*. ($45.00) Available from the Marketing Department, City of Hope Medical Center, 1500 East Duarte Road, Duarte, CA 91010-0269.

Directory of Pain Management Facilities. 1994. (members, $25.00; nonmembers, $40.00) Available from the American Pain Society, 5700 Old Orchard Road, First Floor, Skokie, IL 60077. Tel.: 708-966-5595.

Home Care Guide for Cancer: How to Care for Family and Friends at Home. By P. S. Houts (ed.). 1994. (approximately $22.00) Available from the American College of Physicians, Philadelphia. Tel.: 215-351-2600 or 800-523-1546.

Making Cancer Less Painful: A Handbook for Parents. By Patrick McGrath, G. Allen Finley, and Catherine Turner. 1992. (60 pages; free) Available from the Izaak Killam Children's Hospital and Dalhousie University, Halifax, Nova Scotia, Canada B3H 4J1.

Oral Morphine: Information for Patients, Families and Friends. By Robert Twycross and Sylvia Lack. 1991. Beaconsfield Publishers Ltd. Beaconsfield, Bucks, England. (24 pages; free) Available from Roxane Laboratories, P.O. Box 16532, Columbus, OH 43216.

Roxane Laboratories sponsors the Roxane Pain Institute, which offers free information, services, and materials to professionals and the public, including assessment tools, booklets, and journal articles. Tel.: 800-335-9100.

Partners Against Pain Comfort Assessment Journal. 1993. Iowa Cancer Pain Relief Initiative, Iowa City, Iowa 52244. (approximately 20 pages and worksheets; free) Available through the Purdue Frederick Company. Ask your health care provider or pharmacist to contact the Purdue Frederick representative. Partners Against Pain is a program of the Purdue Frederick Company and Purdue Pharma in Norwalk, Connecticut. The program provides a range of products, free materials, and services to assist health professionals in their work relieving cancer pain. Patient education materials include *Home Care of the Hospice Patient, Pain Management Dosing Instructions, Up-to-Date Answers to Questions About Measuring Pain,* a handout of assessment tools, and others. Health care providers can receive materials free of charge by contacting the Purdue Frederick representative.

Relieving Pain. By Ronald Dubner and Mitchell Max. 1988. National Institutes of Health. (free) Available from the Office of Cancer Communications. Tel.: 800-4-CANCER.

You Don't Have to Suffer: A Complete Guide to Relieving Pain for Patients and Their Families. By Susan Lang and Richard Patt, M.D. 1994. (366 pages; $25.00) Available from Oxford University Press, New York.

Videotapes

Cancer Pain Control: Winning the Battle (12 and 1/2 minutes) and *Cancer Pain Control: Controlling Your Cancer Pain* (12 minutes). Wisconsin Cancer Pain Initiative and others. 1990. ($59 each or both for $99) Available through Marshfield Video Network, 1000 North Oak Avenue, Marshfield, WI 54449.

Helping to Control Cancer Pain. 1993. Available from the Purdue Frederick Company, Norwalk, CT 06850-3560. Free to health care professionals from Purdue Frederick representatives. Ask a doctor, nurse, or pharmacist to contact Purdue Frederick for a copy. For more information, see the listing under "Other Books and Pamphlets."

My Word Against Theirs: Narcotics for Cancer Pain Control. Available from the Texas Cancer Pain Initiative, P.O. Box 980185, Houston, TX 77030-0185. Tel.: 713-745-0957. Also free to health care professionals from Purdue Frederick representatives.

No Fears... No Tears: Children with Cancer Coping with Pain (28 minutes). Canadian Cancer Society. Available from Promotion Services, Canadian Cancer Society, B/C Yukon Division, 955 West Broadway, Vancouver, British Columbia, Canada V5Z 3X8. Or ask your local American Cancer Society if it is available for preview.

Fax and Internet Resources

Fax

Cancer FAX (National Cancer Institute), Tel.: 301-402-5874. Dial fax number, listen and select either English or Spanish, and follow instructions for the information you want. You will receive information on your fax machine immediately.

Internet

http://www.access.digex.net/~mkragen/cansearch.html
This accesses Cansearch, a guide to cancer resources from the National Coalition for Cancer Survivorship. This guide gives detailed instructions for searching the Internet for cancer-related information. It provides information to access CancerNet, OncoLink, and others. Cansearch is continually updated and is a good place to look for new resources.

http://www.cancer.org
This address gets to the American Cancer Society home page, which includes general information on cancer, the

Breast Cancer Network, and the Great American Smokeout. By clicking on a map of the United States, you will be connected to information about the American Cancer Society in the state you select. State access is now available in eleven states and will spread rapidly to other states.

http://www.dejanews.com
This accesses a search of various news groups. Type "cancer pain" at the prompt in the opening menu.

http://www.liszt.com
This accesses numerous lists. Type "cancer" at the prompt in the opening menu.

http://www.Roxane.com
This address provides access to the Roxane Pain Institute and Roxane Laboratories. The institute provides *Patient FAQ* (Frequently Asked Questions), newsletters, clinical articles, and educational materials on cancer and AIDS pain management. The Agency for Health Care Policy and Research cancer pain management guidelines are also available through this site.

CANCERNET
CANCERNET provides extensive cancer-related information. To use CANCERNET, send an electronic mail message to **cancernet@icicb.nci.nih.gov** with the word "help" in the body of the message. Additional instructions and a complete contents list will be electronically mailed to you in about 10 minutes. CANCERNET is also available on several gopher servers, including the National Institutes of Health gopher at **gopher.nih.gov**, and through several World Wide Web servers.

ONCOLINK
ONCOLINK is accessible using both gopher and World Wide Web software. The World Wide Web address is

http://cancer.med.upenn.edu/. Using gopher, point your gopher client software to **gopher://cancer.med.upenn.edu:80**.

USENET
USENET is a distributed computer information service used by some "hosts" on the Internet. The USENET newsgroup named **alt.support.cancer** provides a forum for people with cancer and some physicians to exchange information and advice.

Other Organizations

State Cancer Pain Initiatives

Nearly all fifty states have cancer pain initiatives. These organizations are volunteer grassroots groups of people interested in improving cancer pain control in their own states and throughout the country. Cancer Pain Initiatives have information, resources, and networks to assist with cancer pain control. Education, public and professional speaking about cancer pain control, printed materials, and information make up many initiative activities. Most state initiatives include health professionals such as nurses, doctors, pharmacists, and social workers. Other volunteers are people with cancer, their families, legislators, state workers, and anyone interested in the work of the group. Many state initiatives are in contact with or work with state divisions of the American Cancer Society. For the address of the cancer pain initiative in your state, call the American Cancer Society (in your local phone book) or call the Wisconsin Cancer Pain Initiative (608-262-0978).

Comprehensive Cancer Centers

Comprehensive cancer centers usually have cancer pain resources. For the name of a comprehensive cancer center near you, call the Office of Cancer Communications of the National Cancer Institute at 1-800-4-CANCER.

American Pain Society
P.O. Box 186 (5700 Old Orchard Road, First Floor)
Skokie, IL 60076-0186
Tel.: 708-966-5595

International Association for the Study of Pain
909 NE 43rd Street, Room 306
Seattle, WA 98105-6020
Tel.: 206-547-6409

IASP publishes a variety of pain-control resources including the *Core Curriculum for Professional Education in Pain*, 1995.

National Hospice Organization
1901 N. Monroe Street, Suite 901
Arlington, VA 22209
Tel.: 800-658-8898

Mayday Pain Resource Center
1500 E. Duarte Road
Duarte, CA 91010

The Mayday Pain Resource Center is a clearinghouse for resources about cancer pain control serving health care professionals and the public. Some resources are free; most are available for $2.00 per copy.

Oncology Nursing Society
501 Holiday Drive
Pittsburgh, PA 15220-2749
Tel.: 412-921-7373   Fax: 412-921-6565

ONS is a national volunteer professional organization for cancer nurses with more than 25,000 members. *The ONS Position Paper on Cancer Pain*, published in 1991, has four purposes: (1) to call attention to the problem of unrelieved cancer pain; (2) to define the responsibilities of registered nurses and describe the scope of practice of nurses related to cancer pain control; (3) to support efforts of nurses in improving cancer pain control; and (4) to provide direction to clinicians, educators, researchers, and administrators in their efforts to control cancer pain (46 pages; $6 members, $7 nonmembers). The position paper was also published in *Oncology Nursing Forum*, Volume 17, 1990.

ONS identifies pain control as a research, clinical practice, and education priority. ONS also has a Special Interest Group (SIG) for cancer nurses interested in networking about pain control issues.

American Society of Clinical Oncology
435 N. Michigan Avenue, Suite 1717
Chicago, IL 60611
Tel.: 312-644-0828   Fax: 312-644-8557

ASCO is a national organization for cancer doctors. In 1992, ASCO published the *Cancer Pain Assessment and Treatment Curriculum Guidelines* to help formally educate cancer doctors about cancer pain management. The guide reflects ASCO's commitment to providing optimal pain relief for people with cancer. The curriculum was also published in the *Journal of Clinical Oncology*, December 1992.

American Cancer Society

The ACS has a strong interest in cancer pain control. In addition to publications, the ACS put together the Cancer Pain Advisory Group, made up of health professionals who are experts in pain management. The group assists the ACS with activities related to cancer pain management. Local divisions are sources of information, advocacy, and support for cancer pain relief. Check the phone book for the address of the ACS division or unit near you.

World Health Organization
1211 Geneva 27, Switzerland

For publications in the United States:
WHO Publications Center USA
49 Sheridan Avenue
Albany, NY 12210

The WHO is part of the United Nations and is responsible for international health matters and public health. The WHO identifies unrelieved cancer pain as a worldwide public health problem and pain and symptom control as priorities. The WHO publishes books, reports, and pamphlets about cancer pain control and coordinates a network of collaborating centers throughout the world to assist with its work. These health care facilities work with the WHO Cancer and Palliative Care Unit to improve pain, symptom management, and care at the end of life. Two of the seven WHO collaborating centers are in the United States; one is in Canada. They are the Pain Service at Memorial Sloan-Kettering Hospital in New York City; the Collaborating Center for Symptom Evaluation in Madison, Wisconsin; and St. Boniface General Hospital Research Center in Winnepeg, Manitoba, Canada.

Glossary

Action – The time it takes for a medicine to start working. Also called *onset of action*.

Acute pain – Pain that lasts a short time.

Addiction – A psychological or emotional problem causing people to take medicines for uses other than the relief of pain. This is rarely a problem for people taking medicines for cancer pain. Also see *tolerance* and *physical dependence*.

Adjuvant medicines – Medicines that are "added on" in place of analgesics for pain control. Also medicines used with analgesics for control of other symptoms.

Analgesic – Medicine to relieve pain. Also called *painkiller.*

Analgesic ladder – A systematic method designed by the World Health Organization to increase and decrease medicines based on the amount of pain and pain relief.

Bolus – A one-time dose of medicine, a large pill.

Breakthrough pain – Pain that returns between scheduled doses of medicine.

By the clock – A schedule for taking pain medicines regularly by the time of day or night to prevent pain from returning. Also known as *around the clock.*

Ceiling – A limit on the amount a medicine can be increased without causing problems. Nonopiate analgesics have a ceiling; opiates do not.

Chronic pain – Pain that continues for a long period of time unless it is controlled. When pain treatment is stopped, the pain returns. Most pain from cancer is considered chronic pain. Also called *persistent pain.*

Co-analgesics – Same as *adjuvant medicines.*

Constipation – Straining when trying to have a bowel movement; hard, dry stool; moving bowels less often than usual; or having smaller, more difficult bowel movements than usual.

Coordinated care – Health care providers working together to discuss and plan for a person's care. Also called *team approach.*

Discharge planning – Planning that takes place in hospitals to provide for the health care needs of a person when the person leaves the hospital.

Dose – The exact amount of medicine to be taken at one time.

Duration – The amount of time a medicine lasts. Also called *duration of action.*

Equianalgesia – The approximate amount of pain-relieving power of one medicine compared to another, or the pain relief power of the same medicine given in different ways.

Extravasation – Painful tissue damage caused by vesicant chemotherapy drugs.

Frequency – How often medicine is taken. The schedule for taking medicines.

Generic name – The name that tells what a medicine is made of. For example, aspirin, acetaminophen, morphine.

Impaction – Blockage of the colon caused by hard, dry stool related to constipation.

Intraspinal – A way to give medicines into the spinal fluid or spinal space.

Intraventricular – A way to give medicines into a pocket or ventricle in the brain.

Metastasis – Spread of a primary cancer to other areas of the body including organs and bones. Pain caused by metastasis to bones is the most common cause of pain in people with cancer.

Milligram – A measure of mass in the metric system that equals one thousandth of a gram. One gram is one twenty-eighth of an ounce. Abbreviated mg.

Milliliter – A liquid measure in the metric system. Five milliliters equals about one teaspoon. Abbreviated ml.

Mucositis – Sores that form in the lining of the intestines that can cause painful cramps and diarrhea.

Multidisciplinary care – Coordinated health care that is provided by a group of people from different health care backgrounds—such as a doctor from several specialties, a nurse, a physical therapist, and a social worker—who evaluate a person and form a plan of care. Also called *interdisciplinary care*.

Narcotic analgesics – Medication for pain relief with ingredients related to opium. Also called *opiates* and *opioids*.

Neuropathic pain – Pain that occurs when nerves are affected or damaged.

Nociceptive pain – Pain caused by tissue or organ change or damage.

Nonnarcotic analgesics – Medicines that are used for relief of mild pain and sometimes with other medicines for strong pain. Many can be purchased without a prescription. Examples are acetaminophen, aspirin, and ibuprofen. Also called *nonopiates* and *nonopioids*.

Nonopiate analgesic – Same as *nonnarcotic analgesic*.

Nonopioid analgesic – Same as *nonnarcotic analgesic.*

Nonsteroidal anti-inflammatory drugs (NSAIDs) – A group of medicines that relieve pain, decrease swelling, and lower fever. Nonopiate analgesics, except acetaminophen, are called NSAIDs.

Oncologist – A doctor who specializes in the treatment of cancer.

Opiates – Painkilling medicines with ingredients related to opium. Also called *narcotics* and *opioids.*

Opioids – Same as *opiates.*

Oral – The "by mouth" way to take medicines.

Parenteral – Way to give medicines, including intravenous (IV), subcutaneous (SQ, Sub-Q, or SC), and intramuscular (IM).

Patient-controlled analgesia (PCA) – A way to give pain medicines that gives the patient control. Usually used to manage pain after surgery and breakthrough pain.

Peripheral neuropathy – Pain, tingling feelings, numbness, and loss of function that can follow use of some cancer drugs.

Peristaltic stimulant – Medicines that move bowel movements through the gut faster by increasing bowel motility. Can be combined with stool softener.

Physical dependence – A physical (biologic) condition that happens over time when taking opiate medicines. If the medicine is stopped quickly, physical symptoms of withdrawal will occur. This can be avoided by slowly lowering the dose of medicine. Also called *dependence.* This is *not* the same as addiction.

Plexopathy – Pain produced when tumor or scar tissue puts pressure on a bundle of nerves (a plexus).

Prescription – A legal paper that tells a pharmacist exactly what medication to give a person with directions about how to take the medicine. Opiate analgesics require a prescription. Some nonopiate analgesics require a prescription; some do not.

Pressure sore – A skin sore that results from prolonged pressure over bony points, such as the hip, tailbone, heel, and elbow. Also called *bed sore* and *pressure ulcer.*

PRN – Latin abbreviation for "as needed" or "as necessary" that indicates that medicine is to be taken only when pain returns.

Rectal – A way to take medicine: the medicine is placed into the rectum.

Reflex sympathetic dystrophy – A problem that occurs after trauma, such as injury or surgery, that alters nerve function and results in pain and loss of function of the affected limb (arm, hand, leg, foot).

Rescue dose – An extra dose of medicine that is taken in between scheduled doses if pain returns before the next scheduled dose is due.

Side effect – A symptom such as constipation, dry mouth, nausea, or vomiting that results from using a medicine.

Spinal cord compression – An emergency condition that occurs when a tumor puts pressure on the spinal cord. Left untreated, spinal cord compression causes change in the function of nerves located at and below the level of pressure. Can cause pain, changes in bowel and bladder function, and paralysis.

Stomatitis – Sores in the mouth or throat that may be caused by chemotherapy or radiation treatment to the mouth and throat area.

Stool softener – Medicine that softens bowel movements. Also called *laxative,* and *cathartic.* Can be combined with peristaltic stimulant.

Team approach – Health care providers working together to discuss and plan a person's care. Also called *coordinated care.*

Titration – Raising or lowering the dose of medicine to get the best relief.

Tolerance – A physical (biologic) condition that happens when taking opiate medicines over time. The body adjusts to the medicines, and slightly higher doses are needed to relieve the same amount of pain. If the medicine is stopped, tolerance goes away. This is *not* the same as addiction. Also called *physical tolerance.*

Trade name – The name a manufacturer gives a medicine.

Transdermal – A special skin patch that allows medicine to slowly seep into the body.

Treatment field – The part of the body that is the target of a beam during radiation therapy.

Vesicant – A type of chemotherapy drug that can damage skin and tissues just under the skin if it leaks out of the vein when the drug is being given. The tissue damage caused by a vesicant is called *extravasation.*

Index

HOW WOMEN CAN *FINALLY* STOP SMOKING
by Robert C. Klesges, Ph.D., and Margaret DeBon

> Until recently, strategies on quitting smoking were based
> exclusively on men, but women tend to gain more weight,
> their menstrual cycles affect the likelihood of success, and
> their withdrawal symptoms are different. This program has
> been tested with thousands of women and has had up to
> *double* the success rate of other programs.
>
> *192 pages ... Paperback ... $9.95*

RUNNING ON EMPTY: The Complete Guide to Chronic
Fatigue Syndrome (CFIDS) by Katrina Berne, Ph.D.

> This award-winning book on CFIDS combines the latest
> medical findings and descriptions of effective treatments with
> supportive ideas on how to live with the disease.
>
> **"A solid package of thoroughly researched information
> that, for sufferers, could mean the difference between
> being virtually bedridden for years and being able to
> maintain an almost normal life." —*Natural Health***
>
> *336 pages ... Paperback $14.95 ... Hard cover $24.95 ... 2nd ed.*

THE PLEASURE PRESCRIPTION: To Love, to Work, to
Play — Life in the Balance by Paul Pearsall, Ph.D.

> ***New York Times* Bestseller**
>
> Author Dr. Pearsall maintains that contentment, wellness,
> and long life can be found by devoting time to family, helping
> others, and slowing down to savor life's pleasures. Pearsall's
> unique approach draws from Polynesian wisdom and his own
> 25 years of psychological and medical research. For readers
> who want to discover a way of life that promotes healthy values
> and living, *The Pleasure Prescription* provides the answers.
>
> *268 pages ... Paperback $13.95 ... Hard cover $23.95*

WRITING FROM WITHIN: A Guide to Creativity and Life
Story Writing by Bernard Selling

> Based on Selling's widely followed classes and workshops,
> anyone can create vivid stories and life narratives using these
> techniques. The step-by-step program enables readers to
> explore their lives, rediscover forgotten experiences, and find
> out hidden truths about themselves, their parents, and their
> family histories. The new edition includes chapters on using
> life stories and life story writing techniques to develop creativity.
>
> *256 pages ... Paperback $13.95 ... 3rd ed. available May 1997*

Prices subject to change . . . to order please see last page

ORDER FORM

10% DISCOUNT on orders of $50 or more —
20% DISCOUNT on orders of $150 or more —
30% DISCOUNT on orders of $500 or more —
On cost of books for fully prepaid orders

NAME

ADDRESS

CITY/STATE   ZIP/POSTCODE

PHONE   COUNTRY (outside U.S.)

TITLE	QTY	PRICE	TOTAL
Cancer Doesn't Have to Hurt (paperback)	@	$14.95	
Cancer Doesn't Have to Hurt (hard cover)	@	$24.95	
List other titles below:			
	@	$	
	@	$	
	@	$	
	@	$	
	@	$	
	@	$	
	@	$	
	@	$	

Shipping costs

First book: $3.00 by book post; $4.50 by UPS or to ship outside the U.S.

Each additional book: $1.00

For bulk or rush orders call (800) 266-5592

SUBTOTAL

Less discount @_____%

TOTAL COST OF BOOKS

Calif. residents add sales tax

Shipping & handling

TOTAL ENCLOSED

Please pay in U.S. funds only

(   )

☐ Check ☐ Money Order ☐ Visa ☐ M/C ☐ Discover

Card # _____ Exp date _____

Signature _____

Complete and mail to:

Hunter House Inc., Publishers
P.O. Box 2914, Alameda CA 94501-0914
Orders: 1-800-266-5592 // E-mail: ordering@hunterhouse.com
Phone (510) 865-5282 Fax (510) 865-4295

☐ Check here to receive our FREE book catalog

CDH 3/97